Coping with Caesarean and Other Difficult Births

Coping with Caesarean and Other Difficult Births

Fran Reader
and
Wendy Savage

WITH A FOREWORD BY
CLAIRE RAYNER

Macdonald Publishers, Edinburgh

ISBN 0 86334 019 9 (Hardback)
ISBN 0 86334 001 6 (Paperback)

Published by
Macdonald Publishers, Edinburgh
Edgefield Road, Loanhead,
Midlothian EH20 9SY

Design and cover by Iain McKinlay
Illustrations by Sue Innes

Printed in Scotland by
Macdonald Printers (Edinburgh) Limited
Edgefield Road, Loanhead,. Midlothian

Contents

For Christine and Kate

Foreword

No matter how many important things a woman does in her life—be it climbing the Matterhorn, writing a symphony or making a home—she will never feel more involved in the act of creation than when she is having a baby. And unless she is a very unusual or very unhappy woman she'll want to make as good a job as she can of her motherhood. Women are, by and large, enormously self-sacrificing during pregnancy and labour; they take excellent care of their babies long before they are born. The reward they most hope for is a healthy baby—and for themselves an exciting, not too arduous birth-giving experience.

And for the vast majority, that is precisely what they have. But there are some who do not, and this book is written for them. It's a superb book, solid with information and honestly presented. It tells it as it is, without glossing over the unpleasantness of the difficult birth, yet manages to do so without being unduly alarming. And that is no mean feat.

Like every midwife I wish every mother a peaceful, joyous pregnancy, and a normal, spontaneous delivery of her healthy baby—but just in case delivery turns out for you to be a rather more complex business than you anticipated, read this book. You can lose nothing by gaining knowledge, and you may be very grateful indeed, if you turn out to be one of the five to ten per cent of mothers who need a Caesarean section, or the five to ten per cent who need a forceps delivery, that you did so. Your reading will help you cope with it all—and therefore to have that healthy baby you're working to hard to create.

Claire Rayner
London, April 1983

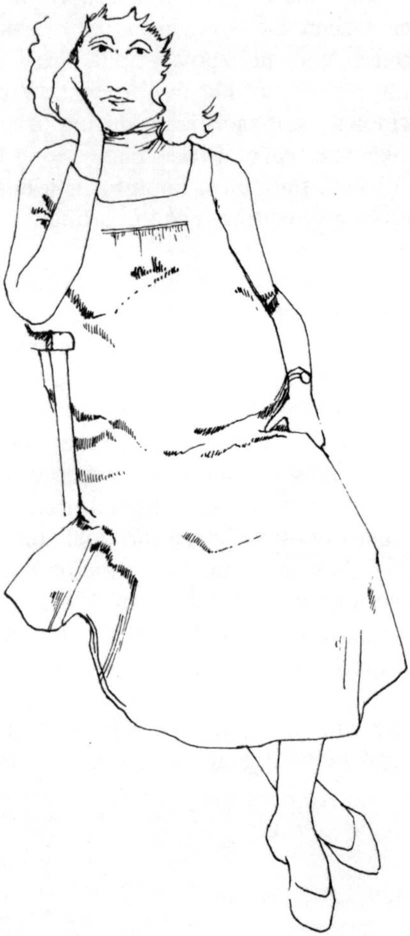

The last few days of waiting
can seem terribly long

Introduction

The birth of a child should be one of life's crowning experiences, the culmination of nine months waiting and the beginning of parenthood. But nature does not always get it right and not all births can be normal deliveries through the mother's vagina (birth passage). Medical assistance with the birth is then necessary to rescue the baby or mother from impending disaster. Between five and ten per cent of babies are born by Caesarean section, which is an operation to deliver the baby through the mother's abdomen: another five to ten per cent of babies will be assisted through the vagina with forceps or a vacuum extractor. Three to four per cent of babies will be breech (bottom) first in the womb; some of these will be born vaginally and some will be Caesarean births. Thus there is a spectrum of ways of giving birth, with or without assistance, and each way can be a success story all of its own.

We hope this book will help dispel some of the fear of the unknown, and give you positive support to help cope, and participate fully, if you should find that the birth of one of your babies is a difficult one.

Every hospital will have different ways of dealing with difficult births and within the hospital it is probable that the ideas and practices of individual doctors will differ. In this book we have tried to combine the ideas and techniques that we have seen or practised ourselves. We would advise you to ask your midwife and doctor what to expect in your own hospital.

The authors are grateful for the help of Gill Mathews, who did most of the typing, and Mary Alexander, Carol Avery, Ruth-Mary Burch, Patricia Egan, Carol Febry, Helen Keeley, Sue Peters, Lenda Poole, Jackie Sanderson, Janet Tarbun and Lynn Woods, who all contributed either as patients or as friends.

Frances Reader
Wendy Savage
February, 1983

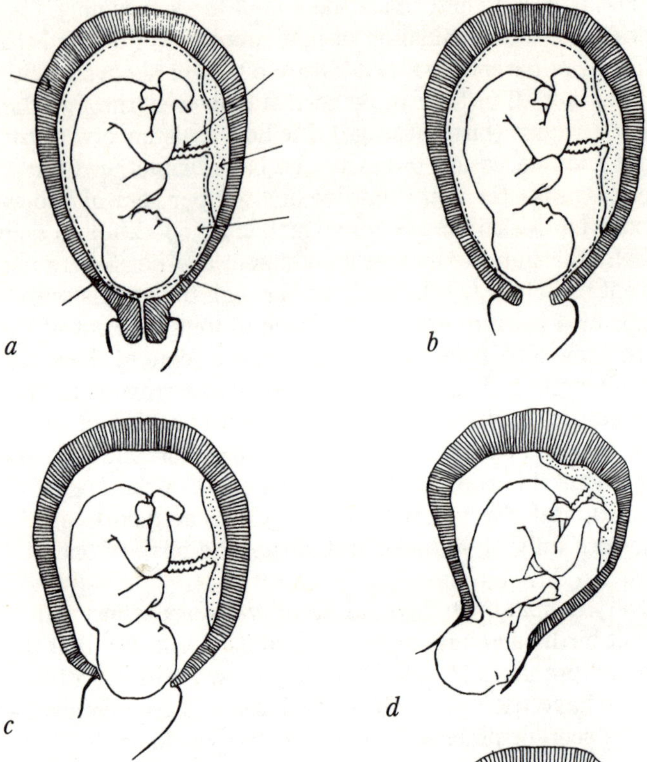

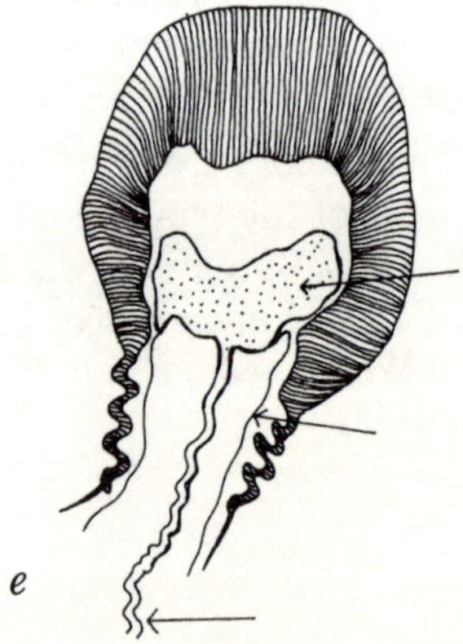

The stages of labour:

a) The contractions start (1st stage)
b) The cervix begins to dilate
c) The head starts to come through the cervix (2nd stage)
d) The head is coming through the vagina
e) The afterbirth comes away (3rd stage)

1 Normal Labour and Pain Relief in Labour

Most hospitals run their own antenatal classes and give you the opportunity to look around the maternity unit; this can be an ideal time to ask the questions you forgot to ask in the fraught environment of a busy antenatal clinic.

Don't forget that your GP may be the best person to approach with your questions. Sometimes the GP can liaise with the hospital doctor on your behalf.

The way that a hospital operates and doctors manage childbirth is always changing; but it is possible to lose touch with the changing expectations of the community, or for the community to misunderstand medical practice. We need much better communication between the medical profession and the consumer. If you feel really strongly about problems you have encountered in the system, then please criticise constructively if possible; or you may wish to praise and thank the staff rather than complain. In either case, you could write to the individual concerned, your consultant, the midwifery superintendent, hospital administrators, or local Community Health Council.

Before looking at what can go wrong, let us look at what happens in normal labour and consider the choices of pain relief available.

Labour is the process whereby the uterus (womb) contracts regularly to open the cervix (neck of the womb) and push the baby through the birth canal. The active first stage of labour is reckoned from the onset of regular painful contractions which also open up the cervix; this may be preceded by a latent period where the contractions are thinning the cervix but not opening it. The second stage of labour starts when the cervix is fully open and the baby passes through the birth canal to be born. The third stage of labour is the delivery of the placenta (afterbirth) and membranes.

It can be difficult to be certain when labour actually begins. Sometimes the waters break before painful contractions start and sometimes after. Sometimes the blood-stained mucus plug from the cervix (the 'show') comes away several days before labour begins and sometimes the show and the painful contractions come together. You should always go to hospital or call your midwife if you think the waters have broken, and painful contractions coming on average at least every ten minutes for one hour usually mean you are in labour; sometimes contractions start by coming every 2-4 minutes, in which case you will not be in doubt!

Contractions are almost always very painful, even in a normal birth, though some women experience little pain. On average, contractions in the early part of the first stage of

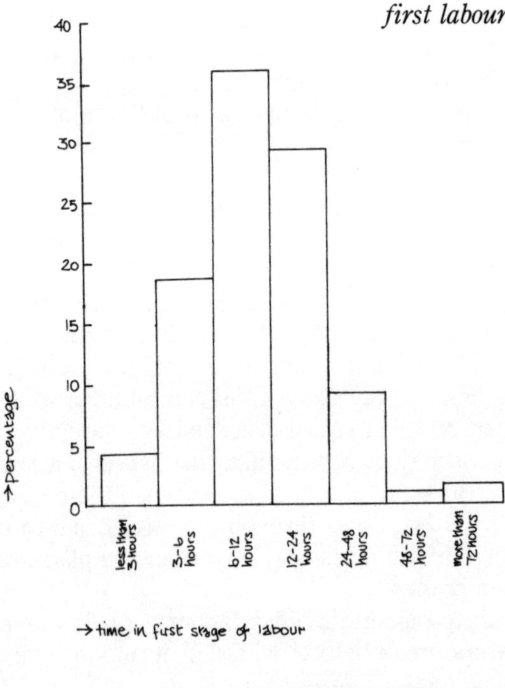

Length of first stage in first labours

labour last about 30 seconds and come every 5-10 minutes. They build up to last 50-60 seconds and come every 2-3 minutes late in the first stage. Sometimes, just before the cervix is fully open, you get a strong desire to push with each contraction, as if opening your bowels; in other labours the desire to push does not start until you are well into the second stage. First labours differ from subsequent labours in that the first stage and second stage are longer, as the table shows. Thus there is a spectrum of what happens in normal labour and there is a choice of pain relief to help different women cope with their individual experiences.

Length of first stage in subsequent labours

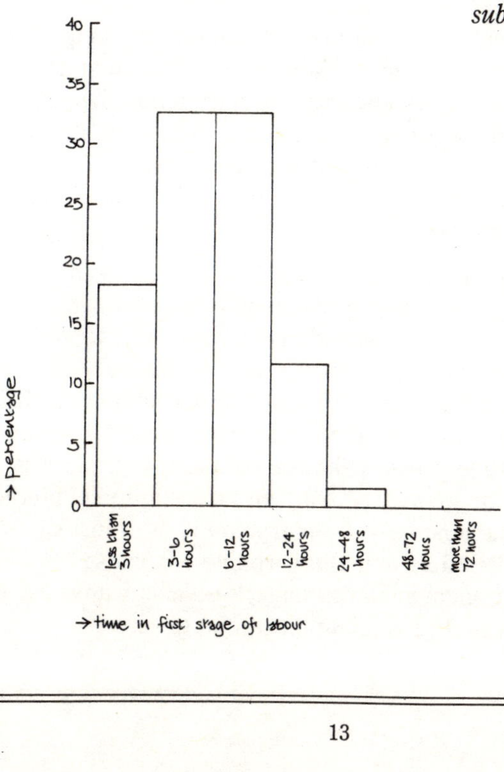

Pain Relief

Preparing your body with sleep and nutritious food will help you to cope with labour. The pain you feel during labour can be heightened by fear, so if possible attend antenatal relaxation classes at your hospital, National Childbirth Trust (NCT) classes, yoga or something similar. You will learn a lot about your body, how to relax, how to breathe through the contractions and what is likely to happen to you. This knowledge will help give you confidence and dispel the fear.

Some women find that, with the support of their partner and/or midwife, their relaxation and breathing techniques are sufficient for them to cope with the pain. If you need extra assistance there are three possibilities–

Gas and Oxygen (Entonox). This is a mixture you breathe, and you can control how much you take. It can be very helpful for the last part of the first stage of labour. It is best to start using the Entonox at the very beginning of a contraction, because it will not take effect for about 20 seconds and this should then coincide with the strongest part of the contraction. The gas is nitrous oxide and although it is sometimes called 'laughing gas' it can also make you cry!

Opiates, e.g. Pethidine. This is an injection given into the muscle of your thigh or bottom which will make you feel drowsy and help you relax between contractions. It tends to enhance your mood, so it helps if you feel positive about having Pethidine, rather than depressed about 'giving in'. It is useful if you need pain relief early in the first stage. If given close to delivery time it can make the baby drowsy, but this can be dealt with by giving the baby an injection to counteract this effect. In some hospitals, Diamorphine is used instead of Pethidine. Both Pethidine and Diamorphine can cause vomiting. It is not unccommon to be sick in labour anyway. If this occurs, an antisickness injection can be given.

Epidural Anaesthetic An epidural is a type of local anaesthetic used to block sensation in certain nerves. It is similar to the local anaesthetic used by dentists to numb a tooth before putting in a filling. The nerves being blocked by the epidural are those carrying the sensation of labour pains from the uterus to the spinal cord and thus to the brain. It is impossible to block the nerves sensing pain without also blocking some of the nerves carrying messages to the muscles of the legs. It is therefore common for a woman to feel weakness from the waist down if she has an epidural. Blood vessels in the legs also open up, which can cause a drop in blood pressure and can make the legs feel warm.

An epidural anaesthetic is set up by an anaesthetist or sometimes an obstetrician with anaesthetic training. It takes at least 10 minutes to get the epidural set up, and another 10-20 minutes for it to become effective and relieve pain. An epidural can be very helpful if you feel you have a low pain threshold or if it is suspected that you may have a long labour (see Page 29). It can be used for delivery with forceps or ventouse (see Pages 53-7) and for a Caesarean birth, but not where a time delay could be critical (see Page 48).

A doctor will put up a drip first and give you extra fluids through your vein. This helps your body to cope with the drop in blood pressure (see above). Your pulse and blood pressure are checked at the beginning. You will then be helped to lie on your side on the edge of a firm bed and to curl into a ball. Some anaesthetists prefer you sitting upright on the bed with your back towards them and your legs hanging over the other side of the bed. Either position helps to display the knobbles of your spine but can be difficult to hold during contractions. Your partner can help you but he may be asked to wait outside while the epidural is set up; if so, enlist a nurse or midwife to help you relax and stay in position—this makes it easier for the anaesthetist. Everyone differs in their ability to perform a task while being watched; some doctors feel at ease but some

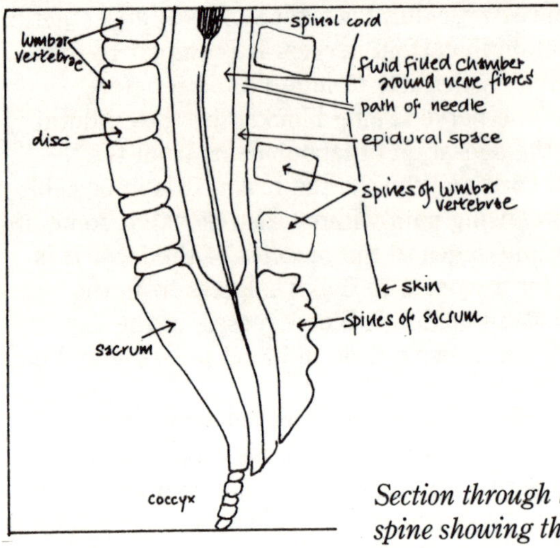

Section through lower part of spine showing the epidural space.

perform less well, therefore if your partner is asked to leave at any stage this may be disappointing but it will be temporarily necessary. Once you are in position, the anaesthetist washes his hands thoroughly and puts on sterile gloves; he/she then cleans your back with an antispetic and injects some local anaesthetic into your back, to numb the spot where the epidural will go.

Once the local anaesthetic is working, he/she then pushes another needle into your back, advancing it slowly until the epidural space is reached. This is a space inside your bony spinal column but before the spinal cord itself. The epidural space is crossed by the nerves as they leave the spinal cord to pass out between each of the vertebrae (see diagram). When the needle is being advanced you will be aware of the pushing, and perhaps some discomfort. Occasionally a sharp pain will be felt; if so, you must tell the doctor as this information is important to help place the epidural correctly.

Once the needle is in place, a thin plastic tube is threaded through it into the epidural space, and the needle itself removed. The plastic tube (epidural catheter) is about three feet long but only about three inches are left inside your back; the rest of the tube remains outside and is brought up your back and over one shoulder. It is stuck in place with waterproof Elastoplast or similar tape. The end of your catheter has a small filter attached to it, into which a syringe will fit to inject more local anaesthetic.

Once the epidural is in place, you can straighten up to lie more comfortably on your side and your pulse, blood pressure and baby's heart-beat will be checked.

The anaesthetist may well begin by injecting a small amount of local anaesthetic called a test dose. Very occasionally there may be an excessive drop in your blood pressure, and this will be picked up by the test dose. No harm is done, because the drip can correct this, but the full dose cannot be given. An alternative form of pain relief or anaesthetic will be arranged instead. If all is well after the test dose, the full dose is given, and gradually over the next 10-20 minutes the pain of the contractions disappears and usually your legs become heavy, numb and warm. You may also experience a tingling sensation and develop the shakes—this is similar to shivering after a swim, but doesn't last long.

A nurse will be checking your pulse and blood pressure from time to time and checking the baby's heartbeat. You may be turned to lie for a few minutes on your left side, then a few minutes on your right side to distribute the anaesthetic effect evenly. If the epidural is needed for a Caesarean birth you may be tilted slightly head down, and if it is needed for a forceps delivery you may be sat upright for a while: this helps the local anaesthetic to bathe the nerves to your uterus and abdomen which come from higher up the spinal cord or the nerves to your vagina and bottom which come from lower down.

Occasionally it fails completely, and sometimes the effect is partial. All doctors who do obstetric epidurals are experienced, but some will obviously be more experienced than others, and even very experienced doctors can have failures or partial failures; this is because the anatomy of the backbone varies in each individual and minute variations in the shape of the spine or position of the nerves can mean that the local anaesthetic cannot reach all the right nerves. If this happens, a second try with the epidural will usually overcome the problem if you are prepared to undergo the whole procedure again—it could well be worth it!

During labour, the aneasthetic effect of the epidural lasts for anything from one to four hours. When the effects begin to wear off, more local anaesthetic is injected through the epidural catheter, and you will again be helped to move from side to side and your pulse, blood pressure and baby's heartbeat recorded from time to time.

It is difficult to pass urine with an epidural because you are unaware that you want to. It is important to keep the bladder empty, to give the baby's head room to fit into your pelvis. The reflex reaction to a full bladder may also cause a damping down of contractions. It may be necessary to have a catheter passed to empty your bladder.

This may all seem as though epidurals are fairly plain sailing; as with anything else, however, there can be problems. If you are grossly overweight, if your back is swollen with retained fluid, or if for some reason you cannot curl up sufficiently, then it may prove impossible to set up the epidural.

Certain medical points must also be considered before you have an epidural. If you are taking anticoagulants to thin your blood (usually because of a clot in a vein or a replacement heart valve) then it is usually considered unsafe to perform an epidural. If you have a condition of the nerves, such as multiple sclerosis, or of your backbone, there may be considerable discussion before the decision is taken.

As we have said, the epidural can sometimes cause a fall in blood pressure. This can be very useful if the doctors are worried by high blood pressure in the mother, but sometimes the fall can affect the flow of blood to the placenta and hence to the baby. As explained previously, the drip can be used to help counteract this problem, but for a short time you may need to breathe oxygen from a mask to help your baby while the blood pressure picks up.

Sometimes the needle goes beyond the epidural space into the space where the spinal column is bathed in fluid. If this happens a dural tap is said to have occurred and the needle needs replacing into the epidural space. Pain relief is still usually effective but if the fluid leaks out from around the spinal cord into the epidural space, this can cause a headache. After delivery you will have to lie flat for 24-48 hours and you will be encouraged to take extra fluids to help to prevent this headache by replacing the fluid. In some countries anaesthetists prefer to enter this fluid-filled space routinely. This is called a spinal anaesthetic; it gives the same pain relief as an epidural, but there can be a greater drop in blood pressure at the time and also top-ups cannot be given, so this procedure is less helpful for long labours.

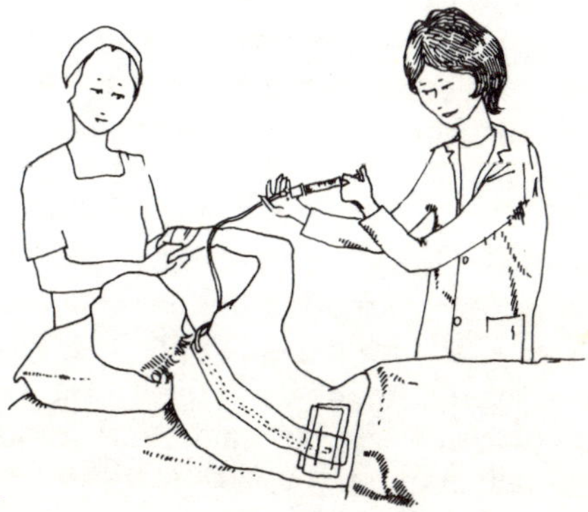

Topping up the epidural

An epidural may take away sensation during the second stage of labour, which may make it difficult to push effectively with your contractions, and you may miss the sensation of the baby's head and body actually leaving your body. Providing you and the baby are in good condition it is possible to let the effects of the epidural wear off as you enter the second stage of labour and then you do not miss out on these sensations. If you feel you cannot cope with this, or if there is a problem with the baby getting tired in the second stage, then the epidural can be topped up and the birth assisted with forceps or ventouse (see Pages 53-7).

After an epidural anaesthetic there have been cases of continuous back-ache over the site of the epidural; this is usually temporary but can last for up to three months. It may need to be checked by a back specialist if it lasts this long. Occasionally there may be a temporary weakness in one leg. It is difficult to know if the epidural is responsible, because similar temporary weaknesses are seen after labour without an epidural, caused by the baby pressing against a nerve to the leg for a long time, or sometimes forceps may bruise the nerve. These weaknesses are always temporary. They may last up to three months, but with the help of physiotherapy, and in time, full power will always be regained.

There have occasionally been cases of permanent paralysis where human error in management of the epidural is invariably responsible. Such disasters are fortunately rare and in terms of permanent paralysis it is statistically much safer to have an epidural anaesthetic than to cross the road. In the light of past tragedies numerous precautions are taken to avoid such an accident. However, an epidural is never the only way out. If you are truly afraid of the possible complications, then you do not have to have an epidural. Your labour and delivery will still be managed by the doctors and midwives to the best of their ability. Relief of your pain, reassurance of your fears, and a safe outcome for you both can still be achieved.

Not all hospitals have sufficient numbers of anaesthetists trained in obstetric epidurals to provide an epidural service 24 hours a day. If you are thinking of requesting an epidural then this should be discussed in advance with your consultant.

2 Why Me?

It is normal to expect the whole birth experience to be natural, straightforward, and fulfilling. Unfortunately nature is not always perfect; what are the difficulties and why do doctors need to intervene from time to time? Medical intervention may be necessary before labour begins. It may be safer to encourage labour to start (induction of labour) before any anticipated problems occur. Sometimes it is better if labour does not occur at all, in which case a Caesarean birth can be planned in advance. A Caesarean birth planned in advance is referred to as an Elective Caesarean, whereas a Caesarean performed urgently either before or during labour is referred to as an Emergency Caesarean. If it is safer for the baby or mother to have a short second stage of labour then forceps or ventouse can be used or an episiotomy alone may be necessary if it is safer to speed things up.

Induction of Labour

The place of induction of labour is still contentious. In the mid-1970s it was performed frequently, usually to avoid pregnancy going past 40 weeks or 'term'. Term is the average length of a pregnancy and is about 40 weeks (280 days) from the first day of the mother's last period. This will give you the expected date of delivery but for this date to be reliable, the first day of the last period must be certain and the woman's periods before that time must have been regular every four weeks; so you can see why it is not uncommon for this date to be uncertain. Sometimes the induction did not work and Caesarean sections were performed unnecessarily, which made both the professionals and the consumer groups question such medical intervention.

Induction still has a part to play but each woman and her baby need individual consideration and the risks of the pregnancy continuing need to be weighed up against the risks of induction. Usually the main consideration is how well the placenta is feeding the baby and transferring oxygen. The baby in the uterus is known medically as the fetus; it needs oxygen to survive. If the oxygen supply is poor then the baby will not grow well. Eventually its blood becomes too acid and the heartrate will show changes which suggest that the baby is in danger—'fetal distress'.

The placenta may begin to function less efficiently if the pregnancy lasts more than 294 days and therefore the well-being of the baby must be checked if the pregnancy is to continue, but many doctors prefer to induce labour at this stage. In some women over 35, and certainly over 40, the placenta may begin to fail earlier, at about 280 days.

If a previous baby was stillborn, or died soon after birth, because of lack of oxygen then the next labour may be induced earlier or the baby delivered by Elective Caesarean to try to avoid the same tragedy.

The mother's health may affect the placenta, especially high blood pressure or diabetes. High blood pressure in pregnancy is probably the most common reason for a pregnant woman being admitted to hospital and is also a common reason for inducing labour. High blood pressure can exist before pregnancy but more frequently it is associated with pregnancy and gets better after the birth. This is called pre-eclamptic toxaemia (PET) and may be accompanied by excessive weight gain (more than 26 lbs (12 kg) over the pregnancy), swelling of the ankles and fingers (oedema) and protein in the urine.

If the blood pressure goes too high it can affect the placenta and slow down the baby's growth or cause the placenta to separate from the uterus, causing sudden pain in the abdomen and bleeding from the vagina. It can also harm the mother, causing fits (eclampsia). The baby may be small and not growing well; this may be suspected if the mother has not put on much weight. Women who smoke tend to have smaller babies and if the baby itself is not quite normal it may grow poorly.

The doctor can check the baby's wellbeing during pregnancy. If poor growth is suspected then this can be checked with an ultrasound scan; this is a method of measuring the size of the baby and checking for some major abnormalities by using high frequency sound waves which we cannot hear; the picture of the baby is produced by recording the echoes. The doctor can also check a hormone in the mother's urine or blood called oestriol; falling levels suggest a failing placenta.

The mother herself may suspect the problem if the baby becomes less active. All babies have periods of activity and rest, but several days of reduced or no activity may be important. Finally the baby's heart rate can be checked with a monitor machine (CTG—cardiotocograph) to detect abnormal patterns, which suggest that the baby is distressed.

Monitoring during Labour

If the doctor or midwife suspects that the placenta has not been working well towards the end of pregnancy or if the liquor (water) is stained with meconium (indicating that the

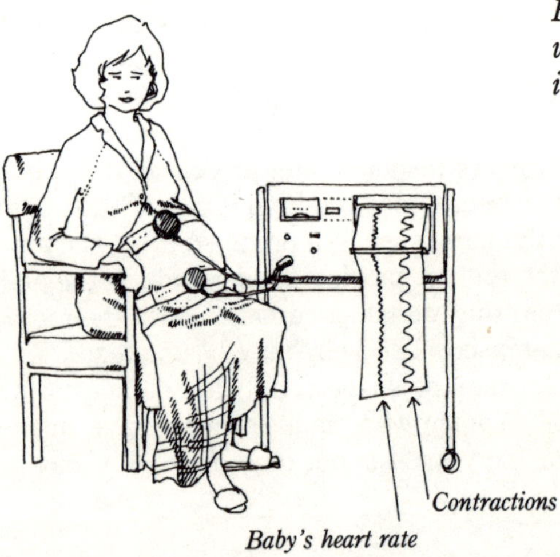

Fetal monitoring while sitting in a chair

baby has had its bowels open, which may be a sign of distress) then it will be necessary to watch the effect of the contractions on the baby's heart rate throughout labour. During each contraction the amount of oxygen reaching the baby is reduced, so as labour progresses the baby may become distressed. Some doctors favour monitoring all labours unless the mother expressly requests otherwise; this is because occasionally the most straightforward pregnancy and labour can lead to fetal distress if, for example, the cord is around the baby's neck.

Unfortunately, monitoring the baby's heart beat is associated with lying in bed attached to wires and machines. If this is necessary you can help yourself by keeping as upright as possible, either propped up in bed or sitting out in a chair. If you want to be flatter it is important to lie on one side or the other as this will keep the weight of the uterus off the main vessels in your body carrying oxygen to the placenta, and it also helps improve the quality of the contractions in a similar way to being upright. Some hospitals have telemetry, which is a radio wave system which allows the baby's heart rate to be monitored while you are walking about. It is hoped that this will eventually be available in all obstetric units.

Intervention before Labour

When vaginal delivery is impossible or unsafe for mother or baby an Elective Caesarean birth will be planned.

Not enough room for the baby (cephalo-pelvic disproportion)

If it is obvious that the baby will not come through the mother's pelvis then it will be born by Elective Caesarean. This may be due to the size or position of the baby or the size or shape of the mother's pelvis. Women under five feet tall tend to have a smaller pelvis; in other cases the pelvis may have an abnormal shape, if for example the mother has previously had a fractured pelvis, or had polio when she was a child.

Fibroids or an Ovarian Cyst in the way

These may block the birth passage, so an Elective Caesarean birth is necessary. An ovarian cyst can be removed at the same time but fibroids are best left alone as they will shrink, and if necessary can be removed later when they are smaller.

Problems with the baby

If the baby is in danger of dying during labour because the placenta is not working well then an Elective Caesarean will be performed; sometimes the decision is taken as a matter of urgency.

If there have been problems with a previous stillborn baby or if there have been many years of infertility then it may be considered safer to deliver the baby by an Elective Caesarean, especially if there are any doubts about a vaginal birth.

Problems with the mother's health

Very high blood pressure (see Page 23) can develop after 24 weeks of pregnancy, especially between 28 and 34 weeks, and it may be better for the mother and baby to deliver the baby by Caesarean.

If the mother has previously suffered a stroke, a rise in blood pressure with pushing could be dangerous; occasionally other medical problems such as diabetes or heart disease may have given problems during the pregnancy such that the doctors will advise a Caesarean birth.

Problems with the placenta

(a) A placenta lying across the cervix is called *placenta praevia* and will block the passage of the baby and cause heavy bleeding. Usually the first sign of placenta praevia is bleeding from the vagina which can occur without any pain in the abdomen. The position of the placenta is confirmed by ultrasound and then an Elective Caesarean will be necessary when the baby is mature, at about 38 weeks, or earlier as an emergency if the bleeding is too heavy.

(b) Part of the placenta may peel away from the uterus, causing sudden pain in the abdomen and bleeding from the vagina. This is called a *placental abruption* and is more likely to occur in a mother with high blood pressure. If there is only a small amount of bleeding, it often settles and the pregnancy will be allowed to continue and tests will be done to see if the placenta is still transferring enough oxygen to the baby. If the bleeding is heavy the baby may need rescuing urgently by an Emergency Caesarean. Sometimes the baby dies in which case the doctors will try to induce labour and deliver the dead baby through the vagina.

It is important to report to a doctor straight away if you have any bleeding from the vagina in pregnancy.

Previous surgery to the uterus, cervix or vagina

A previous classical Caesarean scar is weak (see Page 40) and an Elective Caesarean will be necessary next time.

Sometimes a woman may have had an operation to remove part of the cervix to investigate possible pre-cancer. This operation is called a *cone biopsy* and it can leave the cervix weak so that it may open too early and the baby be born prematurely. If this is the case then the cervix can be strengthened with a stitch which is put in under general anaesthetic at about 16 weeks and removed at 38 weeks of pregnancy. Sometimes, however, the cervix becomes very scarred and cannot open during labour.

Following a previous difficult birth through the vagina, the uterus and vagina may have dropped downwards (*prolapse*) and an operation to rectify this may have been done, in which case it is better to deliver any subsequent babies by Elective Caesarean.

Herpes Infections of the Vagina

Herpes is an infection caused by a virus which is similar to the cold sore virus. Similar ulcers can occur around the labia, inside the vagina and on the cervix. These are painful the first time they appear but they may come and go and be less painful after the first attack.

If you have had a herpes infection of the vagina you must tell your obstetrician so that your cervix and vagina can be checked at about 36 weeks of pregnancy. If you have no ulcers it will be safe for your baby to pass through the vagina but if ulcers are present it will be safer for the baby to be born by Elective Caesarean; otherwise it can be infected by the ulcers, and a herpes infection in a new-born baby can be serious.

Intervention during Labour

The baby needs help (fetal distress)

Understanding the importance of the placenta transferring oxygen to the baby helps to explain why an emergency Caesarean may be performed in labour for what is termed 'fetal distress'. This means that the baby is in danger of dying during labour from lack of oxygen unless it is rescued quickly. If the baby becomes distressed during the second stage of labour, it can be rescued using forceps or ventouse, or sometimes the birth can be speeded up with the help of an episiotomy.

The pattern of the baby's heart-rate in response to the contractions will change as the baby becomes distressed. The baby may also open its bowels and pass meconium in response to stress. This will colour the liquid greeny/brown.

If fetal distress is suspected, the acidity and amount of oxygen in the baby's blood can be measured by sampling a very small quantity of blood directly from the baby.

Another cause of fetal distress is prolapse of the umbilical cord. The cord, which carries blood (and hence oxygen) between the placenta and the baby, may slip past the baby into the birth canal when the waters break. This can cause severe distress and if it happens before the cervix is fully open then the baby will need to be born by Caesarean. While preparations are made for the operation, a midwife or doctor will keep a hand inside the vagina to make sure the baby does not lie on the cord. Sometimes the mother may be asked to kneel and keep her bottom up and head down (kow-tow position). This is uncomfortable, but can be life saving for the baby. If this happens in the second stage of labour, the baby can be delivered speedily with forceps.

The baby gets stuck, or labour is protracted

The idea of a baby being born through your vagina may seem quite alarming. It is not unusual to fear that the vagina and pelvis are too small, but late in pregnancy your body prepares for labour and the pelvic joints become softer so they can stretch slightly and provide more room for the baby to come through. Cases where there really is not enough room are referred to medically as *cephalo-pelvic disproportion* (CPD). This may be due to the size or position of the baby, the size of the mother's bony pelvis, or a combination of both factors.

Sometimes the problem is obvious and a Caesarean can be planned in advance, but more commonly the problem is suspected because the baby's head has not gone into the pelvis (engaged) towards the end of the pregnancy. This is an important sign in a first pregnancy but not so important in subsequent pregnancies.

When the problem is suspected the size of your baby is assessed by the doctor examining your abdomen and then measurements can be taken using ultrasound. The size of your bony pelvis is checked during an internal examination and direct measurements can be taken from an X-ray of your pelvis (pelvimetry). (X-rays should be avoided in early pregnancy when the baby is being formed but in late pregnancy they are safer.) The labour is watched carefully and most babies that are not engaged before labour descend easily and are born normally. If the baby does not descend then labour could go on and on and still the cervix not open fully, so the decision is made to deliver by Caesarean.

The Face-Up Baby. Usually the baby comes with the back of its head (occiput) facing forwards. This is the normal occipito-anterior (OA) position, but it is not uncommon, especially with first babies, for the baby to lie with the back of its head towards the mother's back—the occipito-posterior (OP) position. In this position the contractions encourage the baby's head to fall back rather than bend forwards with its chin on its chest (see Fig.). This in turn means that a wider part of the head comes through which may well get stuck, leading to a long labour where both mother and baby become tired. The contractions are often felt as severe backache, and may be irregular and inefficient. Keeping upright will encourage the baby to descend and turn forwards, but after a long painful labour it can be difficult to keep upright. An epidural can be very helpful under these circumstances. Good pain relief makes it easier for the contractions to be improved using a drip with the hormone Syntocinon (see Page 34).

The baby coming breech (bottom), face, brow or shoulder first. It is normal for the top of the baby's head (vertex) to come through the birth canal first. Any other position is considered abnormal and referred to as an *abnormal presentation*. If the baby is lying sideways or if the brow is coming first then the baby cannot get through and must be born by a Caesarean. When the baby is coming bottom or face first it can sometimes be born normally. A baby born face first will have a very bruised and swollen face, but this will settle over 24-48 hours. (For breech first babies, see Page 61.)

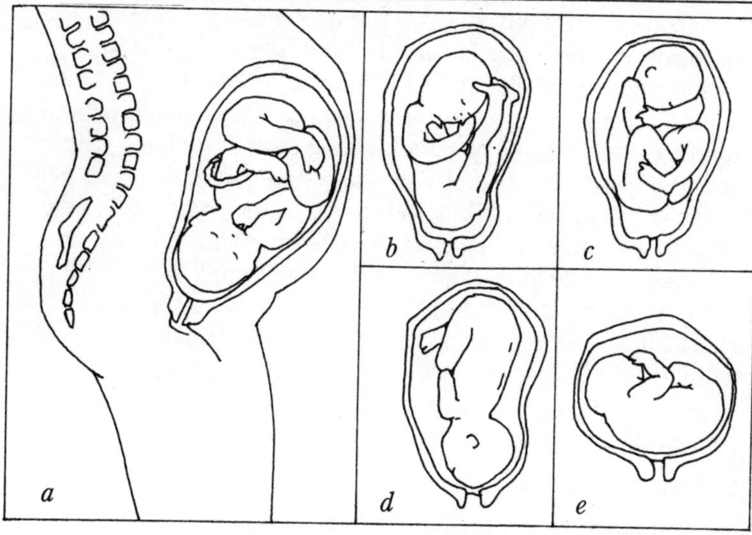

a) A good starting position
b), c) Coming bottom first
d), e) Brow and transverse presentations will need to be 'rescued' by a Caesarean

Poor Contractions. Long labours with slow progress may be due to weak, irregular contractions; this is more common both in first labours and in women who have had four or more babies. It can also occur when the baby is in the face up position. Such long labours can be very demoralising. A drip containing the hormone Syntocinon will help to improve the contractions, and an epidural may be helpful to see the mother through to a normal or forceps delivery.

A Long Second Stage of Labour. This problem can occur if the contractions become weak or infrequent, in which case a Syntocinon drip will be helpful. Sometimes the mother is too tired to push effectively, or she may be pushing really well with good contractions and still the baby does not come. This can mean that the baby has not fully turned around to the anterior position or else that it is a tight fit. Changing position for pushing may help, especially if you can get upright by squatting, kneeling, or using a birthing stool. The baby will need to be watched carefully to make sure that it does not get distressed. If there is still no progress, or the baby needs help, it will be necessary to have some assistance with forceps or ventouse, and the joint efforts of the mother and doctor will usually succeed. If, however, the doctor suspects that the reason for the delay is a tight fit then he/she can either recommend a Caesarean birth, even at this stage, or try to deliver with forceps, accepting that if the baby still does not come easily then a Caesarean will be safer.

A Previous Scar in the Uterus

If you have had a previous Caesarean or other surgery, such as an operation to remove fibroids, or a hysterotomy (a method of terminating a pregnancy by performing a Caesarean-like operation very early on), then your uterus has a scar in it and such scars may weaken with prolonged labour. Labour is therefore watched very carefully to ensure that progress is normal. Very rarely, the scar may give way, and if the doctor suspects this has happened, then an Emergency Caesarean is performed. The old saying 'Once a Caesarean, always a Caesarean', no longer stands; providing the mother is checked and the pelvis found to be a good shape and size then she may well deliver normally next time (see Page 89).

Note: This is not the case with a previous classical Caesarean scar (see Page 40) which will definitely be too weak.

Problems with the Mother's Health

If the mother's blood pressure has been high during pregnancy, it tends to rise even further with painful contractions and pushing, and this may be dangerous for the mother. The doctor may advise an epidural to help counteract this (see Page 15) and then a forceps or ventouse delivery will help to shorten the second stage. With other medical problems, such as some forms of heart disease, pushing can be harmful to the mother and then forceps are again indicated.

3 What Happens

Induction of Labour

Methods of Induction

Nowadays, most obstetric units have prostaglandin pessaries or jelly which, when placed into the vagina close to the cervix, release the hormone prostaglandin which is the same hormone produced by the uterus at the beginning of natural labour. This hormone is absorbed by the cervix and will frequently trigger off labour. The effectiveness of the prostaglandin depends on whether the uterus is ready to start labour. The state of the cervix will be a good indicator; if it is short, soft and already opening it is said to be favourable or ripe, whereas the reverse is unfavourable or unripe. When the cervix is unfavourable, the prostaglandin pessaries may be used to speed up the process of ripening the cervix ready for labour.

Labour can also be induced by breaking the waters and starting a Syntocinon drip. Breaking the waters is referred to as artificial rupture of membranes (ARM). This is sometimes done with your legs in stirrups in the lithotomy position (so called because it was the original position used for removing bladder stones—Lithos is Greek for stone). Otherwise it can be done with your legs relaxed apart, as for a vaginal examination.

The doctor (or midwife) puts on a protective plastic apron, washes his hands thoroughly and puts on sterile gloves. Then he will clean the area around the entrance to the vagina (the vulva) with a warm antiseptic solution. He will then examine you internally to feel through the cervix for the membranes stretched over the baby's head. This examination can be uncomfortable, but there is no need to worry about it. The membranes themselves do not have sensation so the actual moment of breaking the membranes is not painful. This is done with either a small plastic crochet-like hook or a special metal clip with scissor-like handles. Once the waters have broken you will feel a gush of warm fluid flowing from your vagina. The fluid will be checked to see if it is clear or stained greeny-brown with meconium. Meconium is the substance in the baby's bowels and sometimes the baby will open its bowels before it is born, especially if it is distressed.

Syntocinon Drip

In order to put up a drip the doctor or midwife will need to see the veins on your forearm and back of your hand. He/she may use a tight band or ask an assistant to squeeze your arm; either method will make the veins stand out. Sometimes a small amount of local anaesthetic is injected over the site where the drip will be inserted. The needle which goes into the vein is similar to the needle used when taking blood, except that it has a plastic outer covering. Once inside the vein the pressure on your arm is released and the doctor removes the metal part of the needle leaving the soft plastic part inside the vein with a wider end outside. The drip is then connected to the part outside and the whole thing secured with tape.

The drip is normally placed in such a way that you can still move your fingers and wrist: if this is not possible then your hand and forearm will be gently bandaged to a small board, thus preventing movement. A drip used to encourage contractions will contain Syntocinon which is synthetic oxytocin. Oxytocin is another hormone produced naturally during labour. The amount of Syntocinon will be gradually increased until the contractions are coming regularly every 2-3 minutes. The rate of the drip can be altered depending on the response of the uterus and on your ability to cope with contractions; the idea is that you continue to progress in labour and if you need anything for pain relief then this can be arranged.

Monitoring in Labour

The strength and duration of contractions can be felt by resting a hand on your abdomen. The baby's heart rate can be checked from time to time with a fetal stethoscope or a Sonicaid machine. The Sonicaid uses ultrasound to pick up the movement of the baby's heart beating and converts this to audible sound.

If a continuous check of the baby's heart rate is required then a metal disc can be strapped to your abdomen which works on the same ultrasonic principle. Another metal disc can be strapped to your abdomen to record the contractions. Wires from the discs go to a machine beside you which transfers information received onto a continuous paper trace.

Once the waters are broken, it is possible to attach a small metal clip (fetal scalp electrode) to the baby's scalp. This is done during an internal examination perhaps after artificial rupture of the membranes, especially if there is meconium in the fluid. Wires from the metal clip go to a plastic disc strapped to your thigh and then to the machine. Some hospitals put a fine plastic tube up beside the baby's head once the waters have broken to measure the contractions.

Telemetry is a means of continuously monitoring the baby's heart rate using a fetal scalp electrode and a system of radio waves. This allows you to move about as you are not wired to

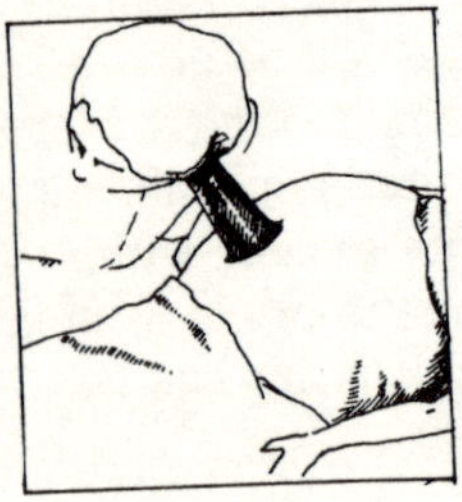

Monitoring the baby's heart rate with a fetal stethoscope

the machine that is recording. This is a new development and is not yet widely available. If the heart rate pattern suggests that the baby is lacking oxygen, this can be checked by sampling blood from the baby's scalp.

Fetal Blood Sampling

This involves the mother being either on her side with her upper leg supported by an assistant, or else in the lithotomy position. The doctor washes his/her hands thoroughly and puts on a sterile gown and gloves, then swabs your perineum with antiseptic solution. A hollow metal cone is then gently slipped into the vagina so that at the end of the cone, part of the baby's scalp can be seen. This is then sprayed with local anaesthetic and pricked so that a small blob of blood flows which can be sucked into a fine glass tube. This minute specimen is then taken for immediate testing to see if the baby is lacking oxygen and its blood is too acid.

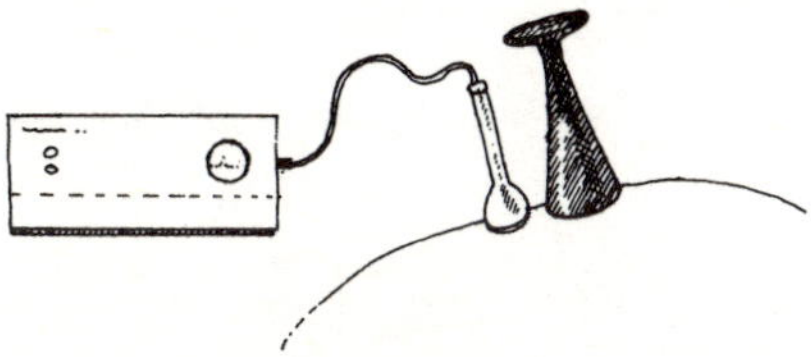

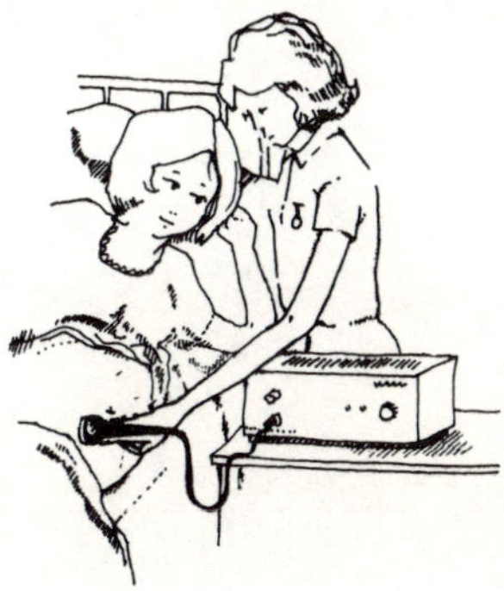

Sonicaid machine

Caesarean Birth

The history of Caesarean birth

The origin of Caesarean section is lost in ancient mythology. The word caesarean probably comes from the Latin 'caedere', meaning to cut. The operation was performed long before Julius Caesar was born, and contrary to popular belief it seems unlikely that he was delivered in this way as his mother was alive during the years of his campaigns. Originally the operation was performed on dead or dying mothers to save the baby, and it is only in the last 100 years that techniques have been developed so that the mother can survive a Caesarean section. As antiseptic, anaesthetic and surgical techniques have advanced so Caesarean birth has become safer, and the incidence of Caesarean births has increased, but it is still safer to have your baby normally. The maternal mortality rate is about 1 in 10,000 for all births but about 8 in 10,000 for Caesarean births.

Alternative positions for Caesarean scar

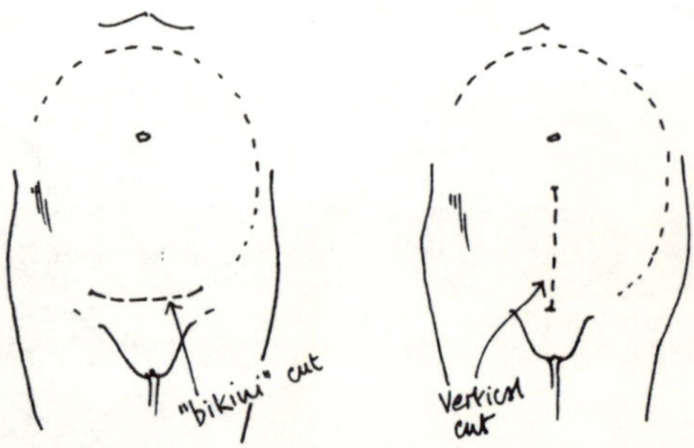

The Caesarean operation

The operation involves opening the mother's abdomen either horizontally (the bikini cut) or vertically; both cuts are about 5″-6″ long. The uterus lies in the middle with bowels above and behind. The bladder lies over the lower part of the uterus and has to be pushed down to get at the thinner lower segment of the uterus. The lower segment is then opened horizontally and the baby delivered through this false opening, followed by the placenta and membranes.

Then begins the longer process of putting the layers back together again. It may take only 5-10 minutes to deliver the baby but another 30-40 minutes to put the layers back together. The final skin layer can be closed by a hidden stitch which dissolves slowly and does not need to be removed, or with clips or external stitches which need to be removed 4-7 days later. Sometimes the doctor will drain any blood that might collect in the wound with a small plastic drain coming from the side of the wound and draining into a small glass bottle. The drain will be removed 1-2 days after the operation. The wound is covered either by spraying on a plastic protective layer, or with gauze and Elastoplast or similar sticky tape.

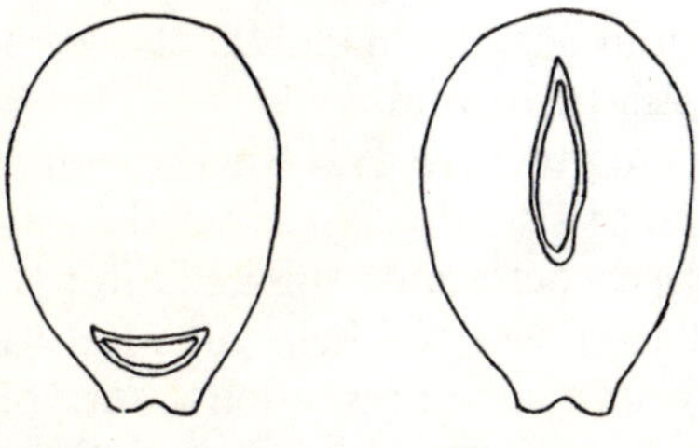

Possible sites of incision:

a) lower segment uterine incision

b) classical uterine incision

Very occasionally a vertical incision is made in the thicker more muscular upper segment of the uterus; this is called a classical Caesarean section, and may be necessary if, for example, there is a large fibroid in the lower segment. The modern lower segment Caesarean section gives a stronger scar that heals better and should withstand any future labour contractions. It is therefore important to know the type of scar you have in your uterus.

Note: A vertical scar on your abdomen does not necessarily mean a vertical scar in your uterus, which will usually be a horizontal lower segment scar.

Elective Caesarean Birth

An Elective Caesarean is one that is planned in advance before the mother goes into labour.

If you know you are going to have a Caesarean birth, then ask the doctors and midwives the whys and wherefores of the procedure before you come into hospital. You may like to talk to an anaesthetist about the choice of anaesthetic. If you know someone who has had a Caesarean section, perhaps she can give you some hints for coping with the post-natal period in hospital and later at home. In some areas there are support groups for women giving birth by Caesarean (see Page 102).

It is still important to prepare your body and mind. The relaxation exercises you learn in hospital antenatal classes or NCT classes will therefore still be helpful.

Once you know you are going to have a Caesarean you may feel unhappy about continuing to attend classes, but the relaxation will certainly help you before, during and after the Caesarean and the breathing exercises will help you afterwards with coughing and clearing your chest of secretions. For your sake and the baby's, if you are a smoker—STOP. It is also helpful to discuss your forthcoming Caesarean birth with the class; it may help answer some of your questions and may also unknowingly prepare someone else who may need an emergency Caesarean.

You will probably be admitted to hospital the night before your operation. It is worthwhile exploring your environment that evening, especially the ward that you will go to after the Caesarean. Make friends with the nurses, find the toilets, and try to foresee any problems that may lie ahead for you in the layout of the ward and your forthcoming limited mobility.

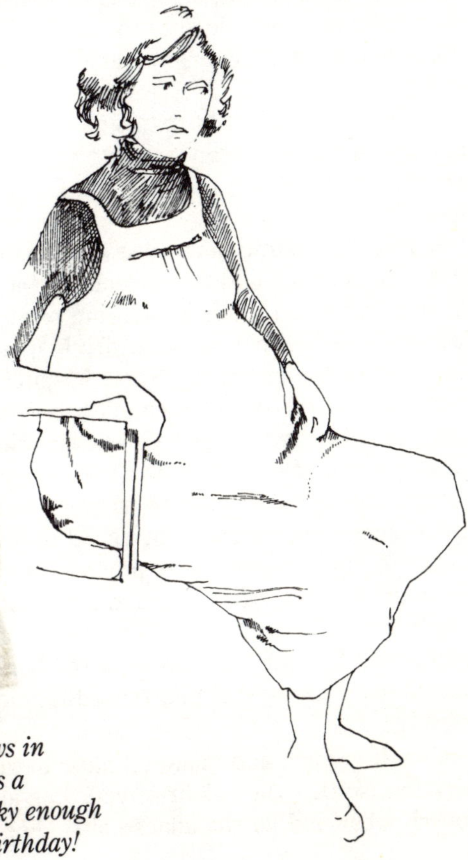

The woman who knows in advance that she needs a Caesarean may be lucky enough to choose her child's birthday!

A junior doctor will come to talk to you and examine you. He/she will then ask you to sign a form giving your consent to the operation. You will also see the doctor who will perform the operation; this could be your Consultant or his Registrar. This is an excellent opportunity to make sure you understand why the operation is necessary, how it will be done, who will be present and what type of anaesthetic you will have. The anaesthetist will also probably come to see you to make sure you are fit for anaesthetic and again discuss the type of anaesthetic planned. Be sure to tell the doctors about any tablets you are taking or any medicines to which you react badly.

If you are afraid of hospitals, or feel you cannot express your feelings easily to doctors, make sure your partner, a parent or a friend stays to help you find out all you want to know.

Before the operation a blood sample will be taken to check if you are anaemic and to cross-match blood for you in case you need a blood transfusion during or after the Caesarean. You will be asked not to eat or drink anything for at least six hours before the operation. Some hospitals will give you an enema so that the bowel is empty and does not get in the way. Your pubic hair will be shaved because the cut is usually made just at the top of the pubic hair line. You will be dressed in a practical but not very glamorous gown and your hair covered with a paper cap. You may be asked to drink a small quantity of antacid liquid to neutralise any acid in your stomach. This acid could be dangerous if you are sick either during or directly after the operation. In a drowsy state you could accidentally breathe the acid from the back of your throat into your lungs: if the acid is neutralised it is less irritant to the lungs.

All nail varnish and make-up must be removed before the operation, so that the colour of your lips and nails can be properly observed by the anaesthetist. For safety's sake, jewellery should also be removed, but your wedding ring can be taped over rather than removed if you prefer.

Some hospitals will give you an injection (pre-medication) before you go to theatre: this will make your mouth dry. You will not be given an injection to make you sleepy as this would also make the baby sleepy. The bladder must be empty before the operation or it will get in the way and could be accidentally damaged. A small plastic or rubber tube (a catheter) is put into the bladder to make sure it is empty. This may be done on the ward or when you are in theatre, either awake or asleep. If you are awake when this is done, practise your relaxation, open your legs and release any tension in the muscles around your vagina: this will make it easier for the nurse and therefore easier for you.

You will need a drip to give you fluid through a vein in your arm. The drip may be put up by a doctor on the ward or by the anaesthetist in theatre (see Page 44). Usually the fluid is a clear salty or sugary solution but later you may need a blood transfusion. Before you leave the ward and again in theatre you will have your pulse and blood pressure checked and the midwife will listen to the baby's heart beat.

A special cardiogram is used nowadays for both epidural and general anaesthetic section, so before the operation begins, the anaesthetist places three adhesive discs on your chest and attaches leads to them so that your heartrate can be continuously monitored.

Emergency Caesarean Birth

An Emergency Caesarean is usually performed during labour where either the mother's or baby's life is at risk. The preparations for an Emergency Caesarean birth are much the same as for an elective, but everything happens faster, which can be frightening. You will probably be asked to lie on your left side; this shifts the weight of the uterus away from the big

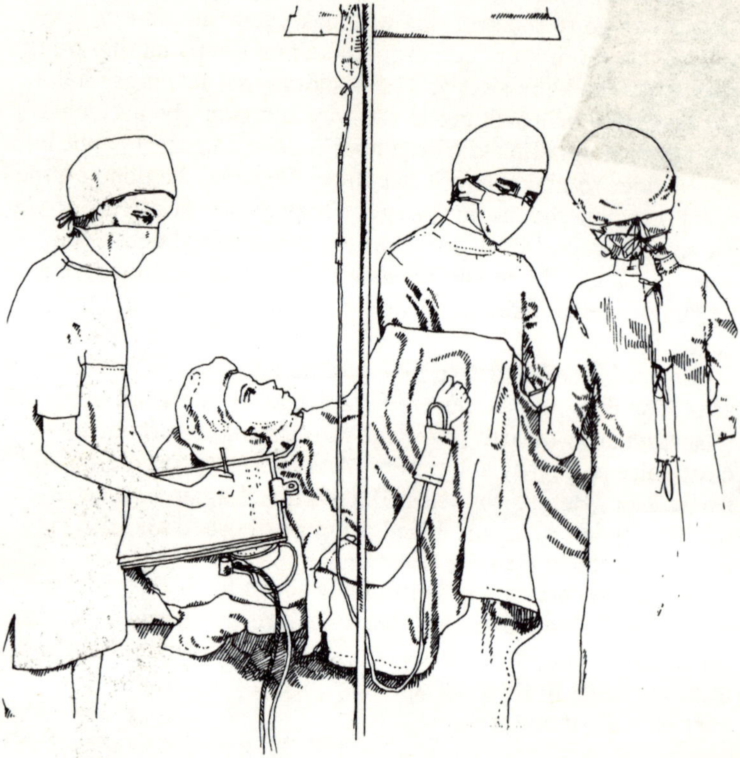

The operator and assistant are working beyond the drapes, while the anaesthetist monitors the mother's vital functions

blood vessels. You may also be given oxygen to breathe through a mask; both are ways of helping give the baby more oxygen.

Usually there is still time for the doctor to explain why you need a Caesarean. At times like this your partner can be very supportive. He will be nervous as well, but may understand what the doctor is saying better than you, especially if you have had pain-killing drugs and are drowsy. It is worthwhile one or other of you making sure you know the name of the doctor, so you can talk about the birth afterwards. Do not leave the hospital confused about why you needed a Caesarean and what to expect in future labours. You may need it explained several times.

It often helps to write down questions before the doctor comes, because he/she may appear to be so busy that all your questions are forgotten in the rush. It is very important for your feelings about yourself as a new mother, and your feelings about your baby, that you really understand what happened. If you were asleep for the birth, then do ask someone who was there to describe events; this will help you to build up a very precious picture of the first moments of your baby's life. Perhaps someone could take a photograph of the baby at, or soon after, birth. A Polaroid camera is ideal for this.

Choice of Anaesthetic

General Anaesthetic. This means that you are asleep for the operation. It may be necessary for an emergency Caesarean, or you may prefer the idea of being asleep. It is common practice to take you into the operating theatre and position you on the operating table before you are asleep. While the anaesthetist is checking equipment he will ask you to breathe oxygen through a mask. This will help your baby; it will not make you sleepy.

Next follows what is called the induction of the anaesthetic;

this means putting you off to sleep. It is the same as with any other anaesthetic, but with one very important addition. You will remember that we talked about neutralising the acid in your stomach.

An extra precaution is always taken at this stage to prevent acid stomach contents reaching the lungs at the moment of induction. As you go off to sleep an assistant will place fingers on your neck, pressing in a special way. This can be uncomfortable, but it is necessary for safety. You will be put to sleep by an injection given through the drip in your arm. This drug passes into your bloodstream and you fall asleep in about 30 seconds. The anaesthetist then gives you another injection which relaxes all your muscles. Once this has taken effect a tube is passed over the back of your throat and into your windpipe. When this is in place the assistant's pressure on your neck is released. The tube is then attached to a machine (ventilator) which breathes for you during the operation, and administers the right amount of gases to keep you asleep.

It usually takes 5-10 minutes to deliver the baby from your uterus; during this period you have a light anaesthetic so that the baby is not born too drowsy. Because of this, women occasionally have an awareness of voices or things happening; this can be disturbing, but the knowledge that it is for the baby's sake makes it easier to cope with; there will be no sensation of pain.

Once the baby is delivered the anaesthetist increases the amount of anaesthetic, and you stay deeply asleep while the obstetrician closes the layers in your abdomen. This will take 30-40 minutes.

It is worth telling the doctors before the operation that you would like to see your baby as soon as you wake up. This should ensure that the baby is kept warm in theatre ready to greet you and not rushed off to be washed and weighed. Inside the theatre there will be a special machine (a resuscitaire) used by paediatricians for checking newborn babies and giving them extra oxygen to breathe if they are sleepy. There may be an incubator for keeping the baby warm, which can also be used to transport the baby back to the postnatal ward; this does not necessarily mean that the baby has problems and will need to stay in an incubator once it gets to the ward. A more pleasant way of keeping your baby warm is for your partner to give it a cuddle and get to know the baby; later, on the way back to the ward, your baby could be kept warm next to you in the bed or on the trolley.

If the baby has been slow to breathe and is needing extra help, then it will be taken away by the paediatrician to the Special Care Baby Unit (see Page 80). Some doctors will allow partners into theatres even if the mother is having a general anaesthetic and then the moment of birth is witnessed by one of the parents. However, this is still a rare occurrence.

As you wake up and begin to be aware of the world again you will be turned onto your side, and saliva sucked out of your mouth before the tube in your throat is removed. As the tube is removed you may cough or occasionally vomit. You will then be moved from the operating table to a theatre trolley or into your own bed. You will be awake but sleepy within 2-3 minutes of the operation finishing.

A word of advice to the partner (this could equally apply to a parent or friend). If you are left waiting outside, this can be a very lonely and worrying time. You may want to be alone, or you might find it easier to phone someone else to come and be with you. It can take well over an hour from the time the mother leaves the labour room until she comes back to the ward so do not be alarmed at the length of time; it does not mean that a disaster has occurred. It would also be worthwhile asking if you could see, cuddle and get to know the baby during the time the mother is being stitched up. You could also be there to give her the baby when she wakes up. It can be a very moving experience to see a drowsy smile as her hand (drip and all) stretches out to touch and explore the new life.

Caesarean Birth with Epidural

Inside the operating theatre you will be lying on the table, literally the centre of attention. A blood pressure cuff will be placed on one arm; the drip is already in the other. A soft metal diathermy plate is strapped around one leg; the diathermy equipment is used to burn small blood vessels in the wound and thus control bleeding.

It may be difficult to recognise people in theatre dress, but you will soon recognise their voices. The atmosphere in theatre during a Caesarean is usually very happy and everyone will be keen to reassure you and boost your morale.

There are usually four doctors present: the anaesthetist, the obstetrician (who performs the operation), the assistant, and the paediatrician (who will check your baby after birth). There will be several nurses with different responsibilities. The two main nurses will be the scrub nurse, who is in charge of handing instruments to the operator, and your midwife. In teaching hospitals there may be students too.

You will also notice the resuscitaire, a special machine equipped with everything a paediatrician may need to help a newborn baby breathe properly. There may also be an incubator or a cot for the baby (see Page 47). The anaesthetist will be at your head, with your partner if he is to be with you. Next to the anaesthetist will be the anaesthetic machine. The scrub nurse will be close to your feet and next to her will be the instrument trolley.

Above you will be large circular theatre lights; sometimes a mirror can be arranged if you wish to see the operation.

With an epidural anaesthetic you will be aware of touch but not of pain and the operation will not start until the anaesthetist is happy that the epidural is effective. He/she will test you with a sharp needle or a very cold spray over your abdomen. Once the sensations of pain and cold have gone the epidural is working.

The Operation

First of all the scrub nurse, operator and assistant wash their hands thoroughly and put on sterile gowns and gloves. Then everyone is ready to begin. Your abdomen is exposed and the doctor will clean your skin with a special antiseptic lotion. Then sterile towels will be draped over you, leaving only a small opening through which the operation will be performed. Unless you really want to see, the towels are placed in such a way as to provide a barrier.

It usually takes 5-10 minutes to get the baby out. During this time you may be aware of pushing and pulling, but not pain. The operating doctor will usually chat to you so that you know what stage he/she has reached. You may also hear a buzzing noise from time to time; this is the doctor using the diathermy machine.

When it comes to actually getting the baby out, the doctor's hand reaches deep into the uterus. This sensation can be very strange, as though the uterus is a deep handbag and the doctor is rummaging around to find something. If the baby is coming head first the doctor may be able to cup a hand under the head and lift it through the wound but sometimes small forceps are used instead. Once the head is through, the rest of the baby's body slips through easily in a similar fashion to a vaginal birth.

The operator's hand is passed into the uterus to lift the baby's head

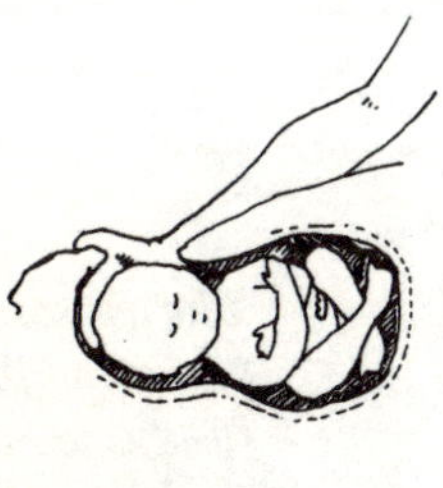

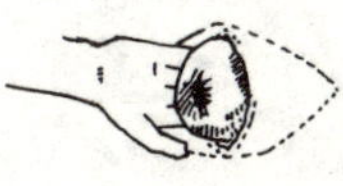

You may be asked to help by pushing or you may be aware of the assistant gently pushing on the top of your abdomen. When the baby is coming bottom first the bottom and legs are eased out first (the baby often passes water and meconium at this stage). Then the arms and finally the head come through the wound—the process is similar to a vaginal breech birth (see Page 61).

The next moment is one of great relief and joy. The baby is born; it usually splutters, gasps and may cry. The umbilical cord is clamped and cut and the new life begins to exist separately from you. As soon as possible the baby will be given back to you, to see, to touch, to smell and to cuddle. The paediatrician may want to check the baby first and suck out any fluid from its nose and mouth. Should there be a delay in the baby breathing the paediatrician will give the baby more oxygen, and sometimes may need to pass a tube into the baby's lungs.

Meanwhile the doctor delivers the placenta and membranes

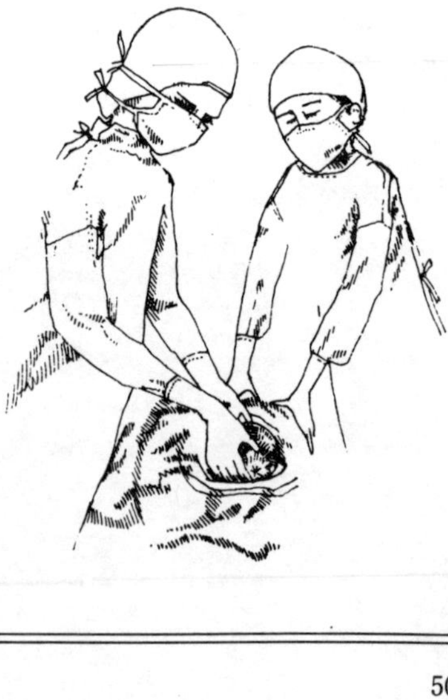

The assistant presses on the fundus to help the baby out

and begins to close up the wound. This next bit may take about 30-40 minutes, which can be rather tedious, and sometimes you may feel sick. After you and the baby have spent some time saying hello to one another you may feel you would like a rest and the anaesthetist will give you something to help you relax or to relieve the sickness. However, you may feel fantastic and enjoy every moment with your baby. While the surgery continues, you may be able to breast-feed; the skin-to-skin contact will feel good even if the position is not ideal for successful feeding.

Occasionally the epidural is less effective and you feel pain. If this gets unpleasant then the best thing is to have a general anaesthetic and this can be arranged by the anaesthetist whenever you want it.

Once the operation is finished, the towels will be removed and you are cleaned up. There may appear to be a lot of blood, but this is blood mixed with fluid, so it tends to look worse.

After the operation you will be transferred to your bed or a

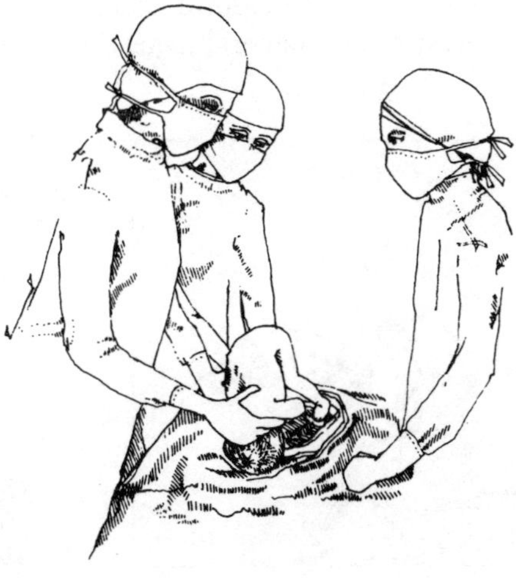

The baby is lifted out

trolley. It is rather exciting to go back to the postnatal ward with your baby warmly wrapped up and snuggled next to you, so if this doesn't happen automatically why not ask for the baby yourself?

Local Anaesthetic

Sometimes the epidural anaesthetic fails to work, and if you wish to be awake during the birth of your baby by Caesarean it may be possible for the obstetrician to use a local anaesthetic. In this case a fairly large amount of weak local anaesthetic is injected into the skin of the abdomen, and then into the muscles and peritoneum underneath. Pain from cutting is blocked, but some sensation of pulling and stretching remains and the delivery of the head through the cut in the uterus may be quite uncomfortable, rather like the stretching of the vaginal opening in a normal birth.

Few younger doctors, unless they have worked in developing countries, will have had practice in this method, but you could ask your obstetrician if he/she has had experience with this technique. As with epidural anaesthetic, if you find it unpleasant then a general anaesthetic can still be given.

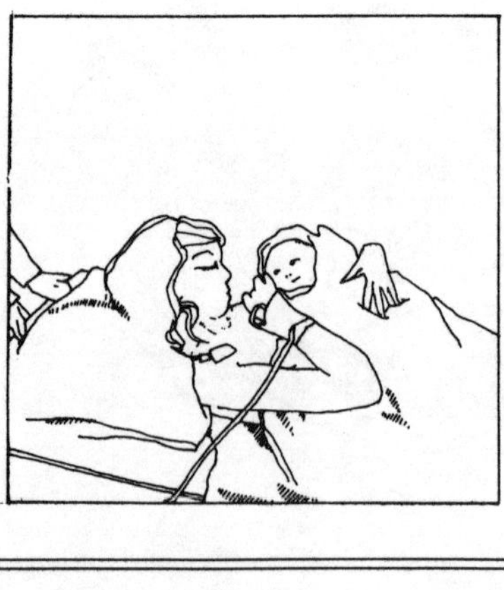

Going back to the ward with the baby on the trolley

Forceps and Ventouse Delivery

The History of Forceps and Ventouse

Forceps were invented in England in the late 16th century by a Huguenot doctor called Peter Chamberlen, and have been modified by various obstetricians over the course of 300 years. They are used to pull, or turn and pull, the baby's head through the birth canal. The smallest type are called Wriggley's forceps; they are protective and pulling forceps. Those used most frequently for pulling are larger and are called Simpson's or Neville Barnes forceps. When turning and pulling forceps are needed, then Kielland's forceps are used.

In 1953 Malstrom invented an alternative instrument called a ventouse (or vacuum extractor) which works on a suction principle and can be used to pull, or turn and pull, the baby through the birth canal. The ventouse has the added advantage that it can be used safely late in the first stage, before the cervix is fully dilated.

Forceps Delivery

Forceps come in two halves which lock together. Each has a blade which cups around the baby's head, and handles to pull on. There are different lengths and shapes of forceps for use in different circumstances. The smallest, called Wriggley's forceps, are useful at the time of a Caesarean birth; sometimes they are used to protect the soft skull-bones of a premature infant. Similar protection can be given by larger forceps to the aftercoming head of a breech birth. The larger forceps such as Simpson's are used for pulling if the baby is in the anterior position; Kielland's forceps are used for turning and then pulling if the baby is in the posterior or transverse position.

When the decision has been made to use forceps the mother will need good pain relief, especially if it is necessary to turn

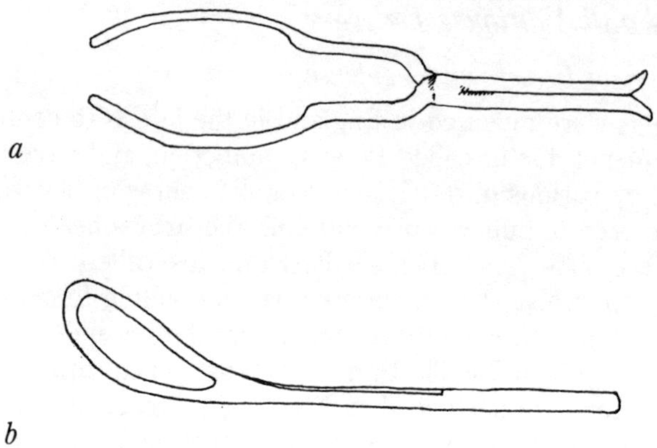

The forceps blades have two curves:

a) the cephalic curve, designed to fit the baby's head

b) the pelvic curve, designed so that the blades fit in with the curve of the birth canal

the baby's head before the delivery. A general anaesthetic, an epidural or a caudal anaesthetic (all of which are the province of an anaesthetist or specially trained obstetrician) will be used. A caudal anaesthetic is similar to the epidural, except that the epidural space is approached lower down, near your tailbone. This can be used to give one injection of local anaesthetic to numb your vagina and vulva for a forceps delivery. More often the obstetrician will use a local anaesthetic called a pudendal block.

It is common nowadays for partners to be allowed to remain for forceps deliveries, except sometimes for those performed under general anaesthetic. You will be positioned with your legs up in stirrups. This is called the lithotomy position. It is helpful if your shoulders are still propped up, both because you can then assist the doctor by pushing better and also because it helps you to see the baby. The doctor puts on a plastic apron, sterile gown and gloves, cleans your vulva with antiseptic and puts sterile sheets over your legs and abdomen. Often the doctor will pass a catheter and empty the bladder at this stage. The doctor will then examine you again to assess the position of the baby and to make sure there is enough room for the baby to come through.

If you do not have an epidural or general anaesthetic you may find that Entonox helps you to cope with this necessary but thorough and sometimes uncomfortable examination.

Then the pudendal block will be given. During the examination the doctor finds two bony points in your pelvis: the nerve which carries sensations from the vagina runs close to these points, so it is here that local anaesthetic is injected. He will also inject local anaesthetic directly into the vaginal entrance to make sure it is numb before cutting the skin, if the opening needs to be made bigger (episiotomy)—this is usually, but not always, necessary.

The forceps are then inserted, first one half and then the other, so that the blades cup around the baby's head and the handles lock together outside. If the baby's head needs to be turned this will be done first; once the baby is lying the right

a) Mid cavity forceps delivery. The forceps blades cup aroung the baby's head as it nestles within the cavity of the pelvis

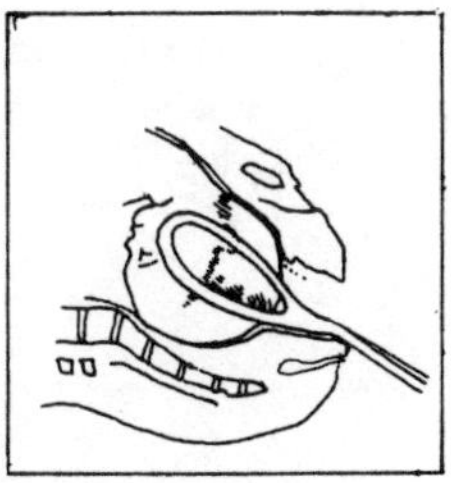

b) The forceps have brought the baby's head down onto the perineum and the baby's head is about to crown

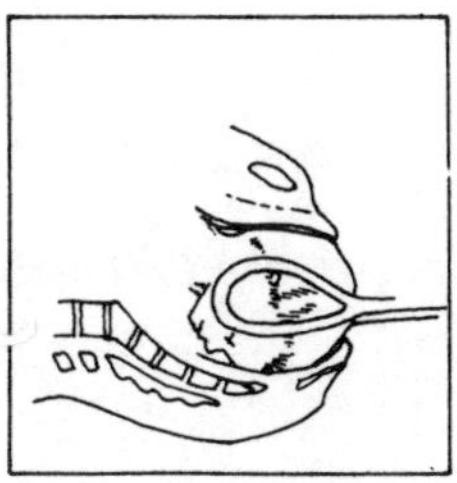

way round the doctor and you work together, so that with each contraction, you push and the doctor pulls. Once the baby's head has come through, the forceps are removed and you can peer through your legs to see and touch the baby's head and, with the help of the doctor, deliver the baby up onto your abdomen. A paediatrician may need to check your baby soon after delivery and perhaps give it some help with breathing, so after the cord had been clamped and cut you may have to part with the baby temporarily. It is helpful if the resuscitaire is placed so that you can still see your baby.

The placenta and membranes are delivered next, and you may be given an injection in your leg as the baby is being born to help speed up the process and avoid too much bleeding. All that remains is for the doctor to stitch up the episiotomy and then bliss—you can have your legs down and really cuddle your new baby; skin-to-skin contact and breast feeding at this time can be very rewarding. The baby may have a long head and some bruises on its face after a forceps delivery, but these go away over the next 24-48 hours.

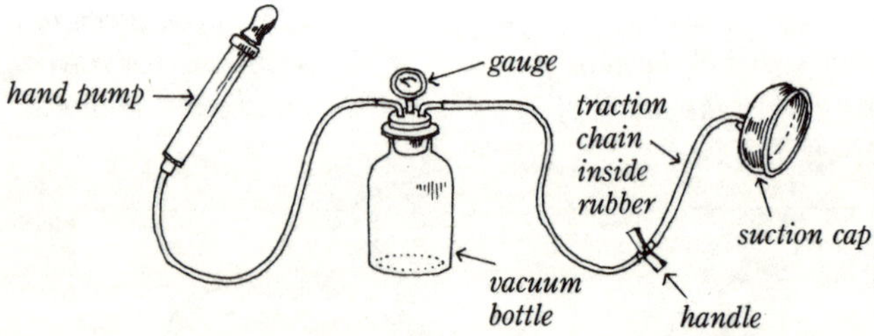

Vacuum extractor (Ventouse)

Ventouse Delivery

The ventouse has a similar function to the forceps, and can be used to turn and deliver the baby. The preparation and choice of pain relief are also similar. When everything is ready the doctor checks the baby's position and applies a metal cup about 6 cm in diameter to the baby's head. Tubing comes from the cup to a special suction bottle placed close to the obstetrician, and a helper creates the suction by using a pump which is like a reverse bicycle pump. When the correct negative pressure has been reached, which takes 5-10 minutes, doctor and mother work together, pulling and pushing respectively with each contraction. Two or three contractions should bring success. After a ventouse delivery the baby will have an especially long head. This is called a chignon (meaning a bun in French). Although it may look alarming, it is quite harmless and will settle down over 24-48 hours.

As stated previously, the ventouse can sometimes be used late in the first stage of labour before the cervix is fully open. Apart from this, the different types of forceps and the ventouse are interchangeable. Obstetricians are trained to be safe and efficient with both forceps and ventouse but they will usually develop their own preferences for coping with specific situations.

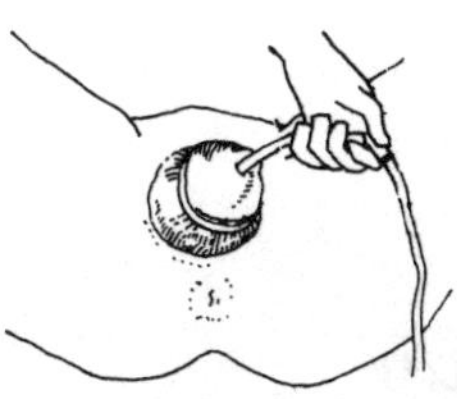

Delivery by vacuum extractor

Episiotomy

The area between the opening of your vagina and your back passage (perineum) is numbed with local anaesthetic injected between contractions. Once the anaesthetic is effective, a cut can be made during a contraction when the perineum is being stretched. This cut is 1″-2″ long, usually on the right side.

This cut widens the opening of the vagina and the baby's head will soon be born.

To repair an episiotomy or tear, your legs will be placed in stirrups in the lithotomy position and more local anaesthetic injected into the wound so you do not feel the stitches. There are three layers to be stitched, first the lining of the vagina, then the muscle layer, then the outside skin layer. Usually the material used will dissolve in the next ten days and you will heal in four to six weeks, but the tenderness may take longer to go away.

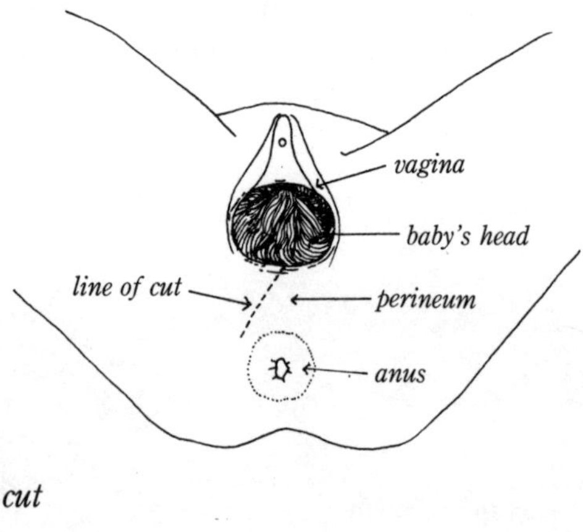

Episiotomy cut

4 Premature Births, Breech Births and Multiple Births

Let us consider the special problems of the baby that is born too early, the baby that is bottom (breech) first and multiple births where there are two or more babies. The reason why premature labour occurs is often not known but it is more common with abnormalities in the shape of the uterus; a weak cervix which may follow a previous termination of pregnancy or operation to the cervix (see Page 27); a uterus that is overstretched, for example by twins; or a uterus made irritable by a placental abruption (see Page 27).

Premature Births

A baby born after 26 weeks of pregnancy may survive with today's intensive neonatal care (neonatal means newborn). A baby is said to be premature if it is born before the end of 37 completed weeks of pregnancy; at 26 weeks the survival rate is about 10%, rising to 50% at 28 weeks and almost 100% by 34 weeks. (These figures vary from unit to unit.) There are many problems with very premature babies because everything is immature, but the main problem is with the lungs. Up to 34 weeks it is common for the premature baby to need assistance with breathing, which may mean using a mechanical ventilator or just increasing the amount of oxygen in the air it breathes.

If you think you are in labour prematurely, you must go directly to hospital. It is sometimes possible to stop premature labour with drugs given through a drip. These drugs belong to a family of drugs called sympathomimetics which means they have a similar effect on your body to the natural response to fear; therefore when you have a drip to stop premature labour you may feel your heart beating rapidly and find you are trembling, as well as the desired effect which is to stop the uterus contracting. If the hospital you go to does not have a neonatal unit that can cope with very small babies you may be transferred by ambulance to a bigger hospital. It is not always possible to stop a premature labour, or even delay it, especially if your waters have broken.

A premature baby is smaller and more delicate, so its birth needs to be gentle. The premature baby's head is particularly vulnerable. If a premature baby is coming head first then it can be delivered safely through the vagina. Sometimes a doctor will recommend an epidural so that the strong urge to push is removed, and the action of the uterus contracting and more controlled pushing will deliver the baby more slowly. If the muscles of the perineum (see Page 58) are thick and rigid, especially if this is a first baby, then the doctor or midwife will perform an episiotomy to prevent any undue pressure on the soft head. In second and subsequent babies, the muscles tend to be less rigid and an episiotomy is not always required. Sometimes small forceps are used to cup around and protect the baby's head (see Page 53).

Up to 34 weeks of pregnancy there is a lot of liquor (water) around the baby, so the baby is free to move and change its position frequently. It is therefore not uncommon for a premature baby to come bottom first. In such cases, observation has shown that from 28-32 weeks the chances of survival may be less if the baby is born through the vagina. This is because the vulnerable baby's head is the last part to come through the birth canal and may get caught by the cervix if the smaller body has slipped through before it is fully open. Under these circumstances, a Caesarean section may be the safest way of delivering the baby, but each case must be considered individually.

A paediatrician will always be present for the birth of a premature baby and will explain to you what is happening and why. You may be able to see or hold the baby briefly before it goes to the Special Care Baby Unit (see Page 80).

Difficult Births

Breech Births

The most common cause of a baby coming breech first is prematurity, but 3-4% of mature babies still come breech first. Usually the cause is unknown but it may be due to an abnormal shape of the mother's uterus or something blocking the opening to the pelvis such as a fibroid, an ovarian cyst or a low-lying placenta. There may be an excess amount of liquor after 34 weeks so that the baby remains mobile. The stretchy uterus of a woman who has had several babies also allows the baby more mobility. The problem may be with the baby; an abnormal baby may come breech first and in multiple births one of the babies may be breech first.

There are various kinds of breech presentation. Sometimes the baby's feet are curled up beneath the breech, sometimes it is sitting crosslegged with the knees bent and sometimes the knees are straight with the baby's feet beside its head. The first position means that the breech does not fit snugly into the mother's bony pelvis and when the waters break the cord can sometimes slip past the baby's bottom; this is called a cord prolapse (see Page 29). If this happens the baby must be born by an Emergency Caesarean.

When an obstetrician finds that there is a breech presentation after 34 weeks of pregnancy, then he/she may try to turn the baby to come head first. This cannot always be done, if for example there is a scar in the uterus or there has been any bleeding from the placenta during pregnancy. Some doctors prefer not to try and turn a baby; many will turn themselves anyway, and those that are turned frequently turn back again!

You may be able to help the baby turn itself by relaxing each day for 30-60 minutes either in the kow-tow position or lying on your back on the floor with a pillow under your bottom and your legs stretched up the wall. Either position helps the baby's bottom to come out of the pelvis and then to turn around if it wants to. If you feel it turn, stand up quickly!

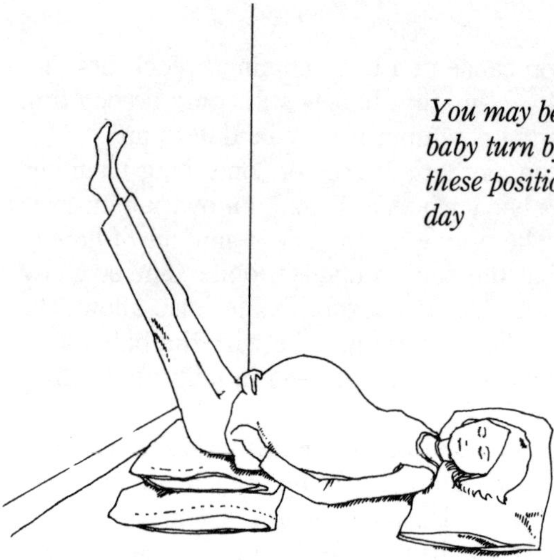

You may be able to help the baby turn by relaxing in one of these positions for ½-1 hr every day

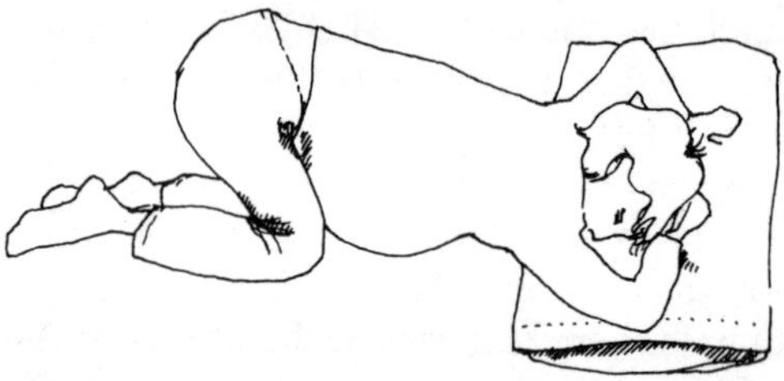

In the same way that obstetricians agree to differ about turning breech babies, they also disagree about methods of delivery. Some favour Caesarean section for all cases, while others recommend a more conservative 'wait and see' approach; if the baby comes down the birth canal normally during labour then they proceed to a vaginal breech birth, but if the baby sticks at any stage an Emergency Caesarean is performed. When considering the right method of birth other problems are taken into consideration and if there is a second factor such as high blood pressure then it may be considered safer to deliver the baby by an Elective Caesarean.

If you are planning for a vaginal breech delivery then the size of the baby, especially the head, will be assessed by the doctor feeling it through your abdomen and then getting more exact measurements with ultrasound. The size of your bony pelvis is also checked by the doctor who is particularly feeling for any prominent bones sticking into the birth canal and then direct measurements are taken by X-raying your pelvis. This is called pelvimetry. The main anxiety with a vaginal breech birth is the baby's head which comes last through the birth canal and does not have time to shape itself (mould) to the mother's pelvis, as happens when a baby is born head first.

Vaginal Breech Birth

You may be advised to have an epidural for your labour. In the second stage the doctor may need to help the baby's legs and body out of the vagina, using forceps to protect and guide the head over the perineum, so good pain relief is helpful and you will be more relaxed. Also, if you do not open up and a Caesarean is necessary, then you can have this done with an epidural anaesthetic. However, many obstetricians (and mothers) prefer a breech birth without an epidural. A compromise can be for the anaesthetist to put the epidural catheter in place early in labour but for no local anaesthetic to be injected unless it is needed.

The first stage of labour is similar to normal labour. In the second stage the baby's bottom comes down the birth canal and stretches the perineum in the same way as the head. At this stage you will be helped into the lithotomy position. Unless the perineum is very soft and stretchy the doctor will inject local anaesthetic and perform an episiotomy to give the baby plenty of room. As the baby's bottom emerges you can tell its sex; at this stage it frequently passes water and meconium. It can be exciting to watch all this happen in a mirror if you can get a nurse to hold one in the right position for you and make sure your shoulders are well propped up.

Sometimes your pushing alone will deliver the baby as far as its armpits; if not, the doctor helps the legs to come out and then carefully brings out a length of umbilical cord so that the cord is loose and not stretched. Then the baby's arms are helped out; to do this the doctor may turn the baby's body from side to side so that each arm can slip out easily underneath the arch of your pubic bone. If you can see what is happening then the baby is frequently wriggling at this stage with its head still inside the vagina. It is left to hang so that the weight of its own body helps the head to come down.

The baby's legs are then lifted up and supported by an assistant while the doctor places forceps around the baby's head to protect it and deliver it slowly and in a controlled fashion. If the birth of the unmoulded head is too quick then the soft tissues inside the baby's skull may tear and the baby may be handicapped. If there is insufficient time to put on forceps, the doctor can slow and control the birth of the head with a special technique using his hands only.

Multiple Births

The incidence of twins is about 1 in 80 births in the UK and the incidence of triplets about 1 in 6,000. Twins are usually non-identical (two separate eggs fertilised by two separate sperms and developed together) but sometimes twins are identical, which means that they have developed from one egg and one sperm. Non-identical twins, triplets and other multiple births are now more common because of fertility drugs, which can cause a woman to release more than one egg each month.

With multiple pregnancies the mother may be very

uncomfortable because of the size of the uterus. She also tends to be tired and anaemic because the babies use up all her stores of iron and vitamins. This can be counteracted by taking extra iron and vitamins during the pregnancy. There is also an increased tendency to develop high blood pressure and the mother may well go into labour prematurely if the uterus is overstretched. It is not uncommon for one of the babies to come breech first or even to lie sideways in the uterus.

Triplets are usually delivered by Elective Caesarean section; twins are usually safe to be born vaginally, but if one is coming breech first then all the precautions need to be taken as previously described. The second twin is particularly at risk and the doctor may well need to help with forceps or ventouse. Some obstetricians will advise an epidural anaesthetic for twins, especially if one of the twins is coming breech first.

After the birth there may be the added concern of the babies being in the Special Care Unit if they are premature or if the birth has been particularly difficult. Then there are problems with feeding. Twins can still be breast-fed with one on each breast and with their bodies resting on pillows and tucked under the mother's arms. At home there can be extra problems with getting two (or more) of everything and needing extra time to manage the babies. A social worker may be able to help provide a home help in the early days and to advise if there are financial problems. You could also contact other mothers with twins (see address on Page 102).

5 After the Birth

Pain Relief

The method used for pain relief depends on whether you had an epidural or general anaesthetic. Sometimes the epidural is left in for a short period and further top-ups are given for pain relief; if the epidural has been removed or if you had a general anaesthetic then pain and sickness (if you feel this) are eased by giving injections into your bottom or thigh.

In the first 24 hours after the birth you need regular shots to relieve the pain; this helps you to cope with coughing, passing urine and moving. Once you are drinking, you can change from injections to pain-relieving tablets. Some hospitals concoct their own special mixtures, usually with a soluble pain-killer plus peppermint water for wind and an antacid for heartburn.

All the pain-relieving drugs are safe for breast-feeding mothers to take. The amounts passing to the baby in the milk will be negligible. It is therefore better to have adequate relief from pain and discomfort than to try to manage without tablets or injections.

Passing Urine

Some hospitals leave a catheter in place for the first night. Otherwise you have to learn to use a bedpan. It may be better to get the nurses to help you sit out on a commode or ask them to put the bedpan on the edge of the bed so that you can sit on it with your legs over the edge; this is more like sitting on a toilet—so relax your pelvic floor muscles and let it flow. If you still have no success the nurses may help by passing a catheter to release the urine and then removing it again. After the first night it is worth while taking time and, with help, getting to a toilet.

Bowels

Your bowels are unlikely to open the first day, but you can get wind pains, which may be particularly severe around the second or third days. Suppositories or a gentle enema can help to get the wind shifted. Do not try to hold wind back; bowel problems are common after all deliveries so it is better to make a joke about it. You may get piles after a Caesarean birth, and if these become really painful special creams and suppositories will help to shrink them and ease the discomfort. Ice packs can also be very soothing. From the second day onwards it is probably helpful to take a regular laxative at night so that your motions are soft and you do not have to strain. Laxatives which make the motions softer and bulkier are best if you are breast-feeding. Bran is particularly helpful. Senokot should be avoided if you are breast-feeding.

Fluids

You will probably keep the intravenous drip for 12-24 hours after the birth. This will give your body its liquid requirements. You will have mouth-washes and sips of water at first, and then gradually build up the amounts you drink, especially if you are feeling sick (retching with a fresh scar is not pleasant). Avoid fizzy drinks; they can cause very strong wind pains.

Food

Once you are drinking freely you can start on solid foods, building up from a light diet to a full meal as your body dictates. Fruit and fruit juices will help your bowels, but do not overdo it if you are breast-feeding or the baby may get diarrhoea. Bran in your diet is preferable.

Coughing

It is important to cough and clear phlegm from your chest after an operation, especially if you have had a general anaesthetic. If you are a smoker the problem can be worse and you risk developing a chest infection. A physiotherapist will come to help you cough and inhalations may help to loosen the secretions. It is worth while making sure that you have some pain relief before your physiotherapy. The physiotherapist will teach you to support your scar with your hands when you cough; this is also helpful when you laugh or when going to the toilet.

Moving and Getting Up

During the first 24 hours after the birth, it is important to keep your legs moving in bed. In this way the circulation of blood in your legs is improved, which helps prevent clots forming in the veins in your legs. Some hospitals give you special support stockings to wear in bed for the same reason. If you are likely to get clots you may be given injections to help thin the blood until you are fully mobile.

Your bottom may feel stiff and sore at first and if so the nurses can give you a soft ring to sit on, but the sooner you can move and get out of bed the better.

To get out of bed you will need help from the nurses and physiotherapists to start with, first to sit out in a chair and then to get to the toilet and bathroom. After the first day or two you will be able to get up on your own; remember to go slowly and take your time. Do not be surprised at the length of time it takes to get out of bed and walk to the toilet, and if you feel uncertain make sure someone is with you. Try to walk upright as soon as possible—you are not about to burst open.

If your bed has pedals that raise and lower it, then keep the bed low so that it is easier to get in and out. It can help to have a 'monkey bar' overhead to help you pull yourself up in bed. To get yourself out of bed try lying on your back, then rolling onto your side; now gradually push yourself up into a sitting position, swinging your legs over the edge of the bed at the same time. From this position you can push yourself up to standing; a well-positioned chair to hang onto may help. The same procedure in reverse will help you get back into bed.

If your baby is in the special care unit, you can see it as soon as you can get into a wheelchair. The unit will give you a polaroid photo of your baby if you are unable to get there. Your partner will also be able to visit and keep you informed.

The Bell

Most hospitals have single rooms for mothers after a Caesarean birth. In this way you get plenty of rest and other mothers are not disturbed in the night by the extra attention given to you. However, the room can feel very lonely, and far from help. Make sure you know where the bell is and that it is in a position you can reach easily when you need to summon help. When you are left alone ask to have the cot close to your bed to begin with so you can soothe the baby; it is very frustrating to have the baby crying a few feet away from you, and when the ward is busy the nurse may not answer your bell immediately.

Sleep

To begin with you will be propped up in bed to sleep, and pain-killing injections will help. Later it is wise to have a tablet for pain relief before going to sleep; your sleep is very important and you do not want a few precious hours disturbed by pain.

The first night you will probably be left alone in your room, and the baby will be taken to the nursery. If you are wanting to breast-feed your baby, then make sure the night staff are aware of this fact, and they will only give the baby water or sugar water to drink. You may feel you need to rest the next night and ask for the baby to go to the nursery again. The nurses can always wake you and bring the baby to you for feeds, or you may feel ready to keep the baby with you overnight; if you do you will still need to summon help to get the baby out of the cot for the first couple of days because lifting is too painful for you.

Demand feeding can be exhausting in the early days even after a normal delivery; recovering from an operation *and* trying to respond positively to the baby every 2-3 hours throughout the night can be just too much, so do ask for more help or let the baby go back to the nursery for a while if you find it difficult to cope. Tiredness is partly responsible for the crying and feelings of being unable to cope which often come about the fourth day after the birth.

Later you will probably be moved into a bigger ward with other women and then it is not only *your* baby crying that will disturb you but *their* babies as well; it seems that just as you manage to get off to sleep, you are being woken at some unearthly hour for breakfast!

During the day you will have rest periods, so use every available second to relax and sleep. If you get desperate at night then a mild sleeping tablet such as chloral hydrate may help you sleep; this is safe to take if you are breast-feeding but you should avoid Valium or Mogadon, which can affect the baby.

Feeding the Baby

Breast-feeding is not only perfectly feasible after a Caesarean, it is to be recommended because it helps the uterus return to its normal size. You may be able to breast-feed straight away if you have had an epidural, or are not too drowsy after a general

Possible feeding positions

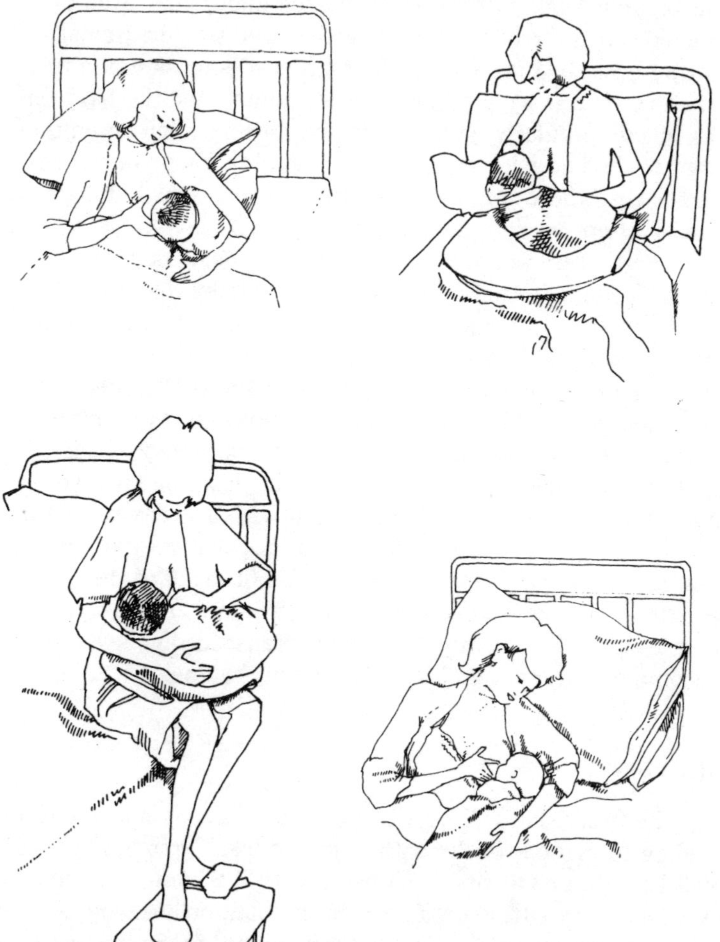

anaesthetic. To begin with you will need help positioning the baby so that it can suckle successfully without lying on your wound. This can be done lying down or sitting up. You can lie flat on your back with the baby tucked under your arm, or on one side with the baby cradled next to you (see diagrams). Sitting up in bed is easier if the back rest is in the upright position; then place a pillow on your tummy and the baby on the pillow. Similarly, you can sit upright on a chair or on the edge of the bed with your feet on a stool to keep your knees higher than the wound. Do not attempt to use the low 'nursing chairs' often provided in hospital.

A nightdress that opens at the front is very useful for breast-feeding (cotton is cooler and less sticky than nylon). A good support bra is important, as the breasts can be very full and uncomfortable in the early days. Your breasts make small volumes of rich nutritious colostrum for the first three days and then the milk begins to come in. This can take a little longer after a Caesarean section, but do not give up hope.

It is worth asking for help and advice from one or two nurses whom you like and trust; otherwise it is easy to get a multitude of conflicting advice and if they are busy you may not get all the help you feel you need, but many of the problems will settle down once you get home and into your own routine. For further help about breast-feeding see the recommended reading list at the end of the book.

Washing

The first wash will be a bed-bath but later it is a wonderful feeling to make it to the bathroom and wash yourself (a nurse will be with you at first). To begin with it is better to keep the wound dry by sitting on a stool in the bath or kneeling. A shower may be easier and a bidet is helpful to cleanse your bottom and wash away the sticky blood (lochia) which is normal after any birth. Later you will be able to soak in the bath, wound and all, and washing your hair is a real morale-booster.

The Wound

It helps to wear knickers that come up to your waist (real passion killers!) rather than briefs where the elastic may chafe the wound. Similarly, avoid sanitary belts, which may rub. Sometimes the wound becomes infected and looks red and inflamed; this is quite painful, but the pain can be eased by a doctor or nurse draining the pus by making a small hole in the wound with a probe. A poultice or heat pad placed over the wound may also help draw the pus out. Salt added to your bath water is a good antiseptic to encourage healing. As the wound heals it may become very itchy; baby oil will help soften the scar and relieve the itching. It is not uncommon to feel numb around the scar; this feeling may last several months, and sometimes a small patch of skin may be permanently numb.

Sometimes a small plastic drain is used to drain away any blood that might collect under the skin into a small glass bottle. If you have a drain this will usually be removed the day after your operation by gently pulling it out. The sensation is one of a momentary aching discomfort rather than pain.

There are several ways of closing the skin layer; some stitches are hidden and dissolve so that there is nothing to remove later. Some stitches are hidden but do not dissolve; these are fixed at either end of the wound with a small bead and are easily removed by cutting one bead free and pulling the other, and thus the thread, out of the wound. Individual clips and stitches can be more painful and take longer to remove. If you are worried about this then ask for something to help relax you and relieve pain before the nurse starts.

Stitches in the 'bikini cut' are usually removed after 4-5 days, but with an up and down cut they will be left in for 7-10 days.

Bleeding from the Vagina (Lochia)

After the birth you will bleed like a period to start off with; this is called lochia. The lochia is red at first, but by about the fifth day it will be changing to be a brown colour and resemble the loss at the end of your period. It finally changes to a watery yellow-brown or pink discharge. Normal sanitary pads should be sufficient to cope with the bleeding but if you notice the bleeding becoming heavier or if you pass clots then you should tell the doctor, as this may indicate an infection in the uterus or that a piece of placenta or membrane is still inside the womb. This can be checked by ultrasound. If the check is positive then your uterus will be gently scraped under a general anaesthetic until it is empty.

Infections

After a Caesarean you may get an infection in your urine, chest, breasts, wound or uterus. If you have a persistent fever, the doctors will check you for any site of infection and you will need to take antibiotics. Antibiotics can make you feel rather tired; some of the penicillins may give you diarrhoea and also make the baby slightly loose if you are breast-feeding. The problem is unlikely to be so severe that you need to stop breast-feeding.

Visitors

For the first day, visiting will probably be limited to your partner only. After this it is sensible to restrict your visitors to close family and friends so you do not get too tired talking to everybody. If you have other children they will also be able to visit you and see the new baby. Some hospitals have special visiting times for children so it is worthwhile finding out the rules beforehand.

This can be a difficult time of separation from your partner and other children. Their visits will help bridge the gap but can also be distressing, especially answering such questions as 'why can't mummy come home today' when emotionally that is where you long to be. If it is your first baby, your partner can learn with you how to change and bath the baby when he comes to visit you. If you are bottle-feeding he can also learn about this and thus have more confidence to give you the help and support you will need at home.

Problems at Home

The longer you stay in hospital, the more disruptive it will be to your family, especially if it was not planned in advance. If there are problems at home then discuss them with a social worker, who may be able to arrange temporary help to see your family over the crisis.

Feelings

Immediately after the birth, the mother's feelings towards her new baby may vary from intense maternal love to indifference and unreality. Studies have shown that about 40% of mothers find that the elation and love for the baby they expected to feel immediately in fact takes several days to evolve. After a long and difficult birth, the mother frequently feels a sense of relief that it is all over; she may be delighted with the baby but her relief and tiredness are overriding and there is no room for other emotions.

Skin-to-skin and eye-to-eye contact are very helpful. A newborn baby's skin is delightfully soft and warm and as most delivery rooms are kept very warm it is safe for you to touch and explore your new baby from top to toe. If the baby has been wrapped up, undo the wrapping and see for yourself; explore the tiny fingers and toes, feel the limbs moving just as they used to move inside your body and study your baby's face. It is important to see that the baby is dry, especially the hair, because wet skin loses heat more quickly than dry. It is very rewarding to put the baby to the breast as soon as possible; this first attempt may not be an instant sucess, for the baby may be tired as well. It does, however, provide an excellent opportunity for the baby to smell, taste and feel you.

Many mothers also describe a time of getting to know their baby and appreciating him or her as a separate individual. It is hard to imagine that the baby that was inside the womb is now the baby in the cot. The baby in the womb was someone you could fantasise about, but this real little person is a stranger you have to get to know, just as the baby is also getting to know you from the outside.

It is common for depression (the 'blues') to set in about the third or fourth day after childbirth. The new mother may find herself crying and unable to explain why; she may be irritable, anxious, forgetful, confused and feel depersonalised; she may complain of headaches or fear rejection from her husband. She may express fears about the baby, that it is abnormal and no-one will tell her, or she may feel inadequate and unable to cope, and sometimes she may express negative feelings towards the baby.

There are many ways in which the 'blues' are manifested; the symptoms may only last a day but sometimes they can go on for a week or two. If there is a real problem, it is best to seek advice and help to overcome the depression.

Post-natal depression needs specialised psychiatric help and possibly even hospitalisation in special units for mother and baby. Depression can be more common after a Caesarean birth; not only is the body readjusting to changing hormone levels, but it is also coping with recovery from a major operation with physical discomfort, tiredness and possibly infection to compound the problems. It can be depressing to keep asking for help and relying on others to look after your baby when other mothers seem to be managing alone. It can also be depressing to see women who had normal deliveries go home long before you; much as your spirit may be ready to be home, your body needs extra rest and nursing care because you have had an operation.

You may feel bad about feeling bad; after all, some helpful person may say, you have a live healthy baby, what more can you ask for? Depression is often a problem after an emergency Caesarean because the labour did not go according to your expectations, and you may have had fears that you or your baby were going to die. You may feel cheated of the experience of a vaginal delivery, for which you had been preparing all these months. You may feel you have failed and not performed as a 'real' woman would have done, and to prove it you think that your body is scarred and ugly. If you had a general anaesthetic you may have doubts about your baby; 'Is it really mine?' or even 'Did my baby die and is this a replacement baby?' You may feel angry with the baby for causing the pain and the difficult birth, and then feel guilty for even allowing such a thought to cross your mind.

This may all sound terribly pessimistic, but these are all feelings which have been expressed by mothers and it is important to express them and face them. This is why it is vital to understand the chain of events that lead to a Caesarean birth, and to realise that failure on your part does not come into it.

You need space and time to express your feelings and medical staff need the time and the empathy to pick up on your need to talk and to cry. Time, understanding and explanation are far more important than pills and well-meaning people saying 'pull yourself together'. Try to share your feelings with your partner. He will also have had fears of losing the two most important people in the world to him, and may welcome the chance to talk about the experience.

If you have no partner to help you, this can be a particularly difficult time. Parents and friends can provide a sensitive listening ear, or perhaps you may value the chance to talk to a social worker; she may be able to provide practical advice as well as emotional support. There are Caesarean section support groups in several parts of the UK and a mother who had a similar experience may be able to see you in hospital or at home. (See addresses on Page 102.)

Let us consider the problem of separation; how detrimental is this to the mother/child relationship in the long run? It does appear that the concept of bonding like glue—if mother and baby are instantly stuck together then all will be well—is far too simplistic. Separation problems are something the medical profession is now more aware of, and every effort is made to unite mother and baby as soon as possible. Parents are encouraged to visit their babies in the Special Care Baby Units and to touch them and help to care for them. Building up the relationship may take longer but with understanding and patience it will develop.

On the positive side, many mothers do feel completely compensated after a Caesarean by the end result of a beautiful healthy baby, and as they begin to heal and become more mobile so the joy of this new baby gives them a strength to recover more quickly than recovery from other forms of major surgery. It is then possible to look upon the Caesarean birth as a positive experience, and to say 'my baby was born a cut above'.

After a Difficult Vaginal Delivery

The main problems after a difficult vaginal birth are passing urine, opening your bowels and sitting down on your episiotomy scar. Sometimes you can be bruised and swollen, so that you need a catheter to pass urine for the first day or two. Passing urine into a warm bath may help if you are having trouble. Laxatives will help to keep your motions soft and less painful to pass. A soft pillow to sit on, or a rubber ring, can help for a painful episiotomy. Ice packs also help reduce the swelling. It is important to wash your bottom carefully after you have been to the toilet; most hospitals have bidets for this purpose. A little salt in your bath water encourages the episiotomy to heal. It is important to keep your bottom dry, as dampness around the wound encourages infection. A hair dryer can work wonders if you find drying with a towel very uncomfortable.

Usually the recovery period after a forceps or ventouse delivery is very similar to that for a normal delivery. You are soon able to do everything for yourself and your baby and will not be delayed from going home.

You may feel disappointment or a sense of failure that you did not push the baby out yourself, but again adequate explanations of the events that led up to you needing assistance, and being able to express your feelings, are important to help you come to terms with events.

You may fear damage to the vagina from the forceps or ventouse or from a larger episiotomy, but the vagina is like the inside of your mouth, and has amazing powers of healing. The doctors and midwives will inspect your stitches to ensure that you are healing normally. Post-natal exercises will help to tighten the pelvic muscles around your vagina and although the soreness may last a little longer than after a normal delivery with no stitches, the vagina will heal and intercourse will soon be possible and satisfying (see Page 86).

In summary, therefore, with any difficult birth it is important to have an adequate explanation of the chain of events, and for the mother and father to participate in the birth where possible, and to be together with the baby as soon as possible afterwards.

Coping with a Sick Baby

If your Caesarean was performed because the baby was premature or was showing signs of distress, the baby may need to be nursed in a special care baby nursery or even transferred to an intensive care unit, which may not be in the same hospital. If you were awake at the time of delivery, the paediatrician will usually be able to let you see and hold the baby before taking it to the nursery, but if you are delivered under a general anaesthetic it will be a great shock to wake up and find no cot near your bed. This may increase the feeling of unreality that some women have about the birth, and this, coupled with anxiety about the baby's condition, may make the discomfort of the postoperative state seem almost intolerable.

Hospitals today realise the importance of keeping the mother informed, and will wheel you down to see the baby as soon as you can sit in a chair. Neonatal (which means newborn) intensive care units usually take a polaroid picture of the baby in its incubator, and send a paediatrician along to explain what all the tubes and wires attached to the baby are for.

Paediatricians now have the skill and the machines to help very sick babies recover, after a difficult delivery, from many of the conditions which used to kill them, and the long-term results are very good. However, this is a very anxious time for the parents, and sometimes confusion arises if different doctors try to explain complicated things using different words. Remember that you can always ask the consultant in charge to explain things if you are worried.

If the Baby Dies

About one Caesarean baby in a hundred will die, and although it is unusual after a planned Caesarean section to have a stillborn baby, a few may be malformed and die soon after birth. Women who have their babies early, or who develop severe high blood pressure or bleed heavily are much more likely to lose their babies than those who reach term, and as about four women out of five having Caesareans are at full term, they are more likely to have a live baby.

The death of a baby before birth may be even more difficult for the mother to accept than if the baby has lived for a few days. Psychologically, birth marks the change from the 'inside baby', a perfect idealised creature, part of the mother herself, and the real, crying, active baby—a person outside herself. If she does not see the stillborn child, especially if the birth has been by Caesarean or forceps under a general anaesthetic, it may be very hard to believe that she really has given birth and to start mourning the loss of the child.

Seeing and touching the dead child helps women to come to terms with their inner feelings and believe in the sad reality of the situation. Sadness, anger, disbelief, a feeling of guilt, physical symptoms such as a sinking feeling in the pit of the stomach, palpitations or dizziness, sleeplessness, loss of appetite and swings of mood are normal reactions to the death of a loved person, and the baby *is* a loved person to the parents. Your partner also feels the same way, but you and your partner may move through the different moods and emotions at different rates, which can cause misunderstandings. Doctors and midwives also feel a sense of failure, and may find it hard to repeat the explanations that the woman needs, but cannot take in or understand. The man usually has to register the death and make arrangements for the funeral, and generally cope with a stiff upper lip, and may feel that somehow it is his fault that the woman he loves has been damaged in the process of giving birth.

Most couples find the ritual of a funeral and burial or cremation helpful in marking the importance of the baby to them, and this can usually be arranged ten days or so after the delivery, so that the mother can attend. If she is not fit, most hospitals have a chaplain who will bless the stillborn baby or arrange some kind of service in the hospital for those that wish it.

Doctors will usually ask for a post-mortem to find out as much as possible about the baby's death, and most parents find this helps them in the task of trying to make sense of the death. A photograph of the baby, or mementoes such as the name band or a lock or hair, are kept and treasured by many couples, and you can ask the hospital to take a photograph if this is not offered to you.

It is only recently that doctors have really understood how seriously the couple may be affected by the death of a baby around the time of birth, but there is now more help available to help couples to come to terms with this sad experience. The Health Education Council produce a very helpful leaflet called *The Loss of Your Baby* (see Page 102).

6 Going Home

Seven to ten days after your Caesarean, you will be going home. Leaving hospital is an exciting moment, but beware—even a short journey can be exhausting. You will need to plan your life around your limited mobility for a while. If you have stairs, then make arrangements for everything you need to be on one level, so that you only have to make one journey up and down stairs each day. You are recovering from an operation as well as having to cope with the normal stresses and strains of having a baby, and you can expect to find life very tiring for a while. You will need all the help you can get!

Sleep

You will get tired easily. It can take anything from three to six months to recover all your old energy, simply because you have had a major operation. Do not set yourself high standards; take things slowly, and rest when the baby is asleep—do not use this as an opportunity to dash around cleaning. Tiredness can blow minor problems out of proportion. If you are breast-feeding, have the baby's cot next to your bed so that you can reach over without actually getting up. You may prefer to sleep with the baby in bed with you. There is no risk of suffocating the baby as nature seems to provide parents with an awareness while they are asleep, so the baby is safe. If you are bottle-feeding then enlist your partner's help for some of the feeds. He can also be very helpful if you are breast-feeding, picking up the baby and changing him or her ready for feeding, so that you can stay tucked up in bed!

Bleeding from the Vagina and Restarting Periods

By the time you get home you should not have any further fresh bleeding, but you may well have a pinky-brown discharge, which could last up to six weeks. Do not use any internal protection for the first six weeks because of the risk of introducing infection. Your first period will usually come one or two months after the baby's birth but if you are breast-feeding then you may not have a period at all, or you may just have a few spots of blood. By the time you have your first period it will be safe to use tampons again, if this is what you prefer.

Food

If you had a planned Caesarean you may have been able to stock up your cupboards or freezer beforehand. Rely on convenience foods for a while, and remember that if you are breast-feeding you will need plenty of fluids.

Washing Yourself

Always have someone around when you bathe at home for several weeks. You may find it physically difficult to get in and out of a bath alone; a stool or upturned bucket to sit on in the bath can be helpful. If you have a shower, this may be easier to use.

Washing Clothes

Your partner or friends could do the washing—and don't aim for perfection! You may only be able to keep up with the nappies some days. Delegate the ironing too, or else sit down if you do any yourself.

Changing the Baby

Find a flat surface at a suitable height for changing the baby so that you do not need to stoop. Disposable nappies can be helpful, especially in winter when it is difficult to dry towelling nappies.

Shopping

Again, get help, and avoid carrying heavy baskets or bags for at least four to six weeks.

Housework

Don't aim for perfection—a bit of dust never hurt anyone. You will need help with the vacuum cleaner, changing beds, washing clothes, and so on. If you find problems in getting help, see if your doctor or social services department can arrange a home help.

Visitors

Make sure they let *you* sit down and hold the baby while *they* make the tea! Restrict your visitors to the few that you know will help, and with whom you can be honest and open. Too many casual visitors who need entertaining can be very tiring.

Toddlers

'Don't lift anything heavy' is easier said than done if you have another child who wants to share in your affections, and who may be feeling jealous of the new arrival. Dads and friends can be very helpful looking after the older children. Lifting a toddler after the first three weeks is unlikely to be dangerous, and kissing and cuddling are of course quite safe. Try to involve the older child in caring for the new baby and give a special cuddle at or after baby's feeding times.

Long separation from any child can lead to behaviour problems. The child may ignore you or be spiteful to the new baby; or it may regress to clinging and demanding behaviour. It is important to include the other child and also to find times when the new baby is asleep to give your attention completely to your other child or children.

Going back to work

If you have a job, you may not feel well enough to go back at the end of normal maternity leave. Consult your doctor before going back—he may recommend postponing your return.

Sex

Once the wound is healed and no longer tender, and the vaginal bleeding has stopped, you can make love and enjoy sex again. Sometimes tiredness and bad feelings about the birth can make it difficult for you to relax. About 10-20% of couples resume an active sex life before the post-natal visit at six weeks. After a difficult birth it is likely to take longer, but most couples are sexually active again three months after the birth. The frequency of intercourse may be less than before the pregnancy, because of tiredness, but most couples return to their pre-pregnancy enjoyment of sex in six months to a year.

There can be problems with sex after the birth; these can be related to pain from stitches in the vagina or fear of another pregnancy, or they can be more subtle subconscious problems because the woman has changed her role to become a mother. It can be difficult for either the man or the woman to come to terms with a sexual mother. If there are problems, talk about them with your partner and then with an understanding doctor, midwife or health visitor.

Local pain or discomfort in scar tissue can often be helped by using K-Y jelly to soften and lubricate the vaginal opening before intercourse. Pain during penetration can lead to a fear of love-making and put further stress on your relationship with your partner at this very vulnerable time.

Contraception

A doctor will advise you before you leave hospital and your GP or family planning clinic can help counsel you afterwards.

The Pill. There are two sorts of pill. The combined oestrogen and progestogen pill is best avoided for the first six weeks because of your recent surgery and the risk of blood clots. It may also suppress breast milk. The progestogen-only pill can be taken first, and is safe for breast-feeding mothers. You can change onto the combined pill later.

The Coil. This can be fitted at your post-natal visit at six weeks.

Barrier Methods. Sheaths and pessaries are ideal to begin with. If you used a cap before delivery you will need to have the size checked as you may now need a bigger one.

Sterilization. Sometimes women request sterilization at the time of a Caesarean. Don't forget that the baby's survival to adulthood can never be guaranteed. Sterilization at the time of Caesarean carries a higher failure rate, so it is worth waiting several months before making such a big decision. Perhaps your partner might consider vasectomy?

Female sterilization can be done in two ways. The most common is using a small telescope-like instrument called a laparoscope. The laparoscope is put into the abdomen through a small hole made just below the umbilicus. The tubes can then be seen and then burnt or blocked with a small ring or clip. The other method involves making a small cut in the abdomen just above the pubic hair line and then cutting out a segment from each tube (tubal ligation). Both operations are done under a general anaesthetic. The stay in hospital is likely to be 48 hours after laparoscopic sterilization but could be 4-5 days after tubal ligation. If you are still breast-feeding, it is usually possible to bring the baby into hospital with you.

Post-natal Exercises

The physiotherapist will help and advise you in hospital; at home, following the advice in the booklet *You after Childbirth* (see reading list) will help.

Follow-up

Once you are at home, the midwife will visit you up to the tenth day, and can continue to visit up to the end of the first month. Your GP may also visit you, and after ten days the health visitor will call. She is a nurse especially trained to advise you about the baby's feeding, development, vaccinations, etc. She will follow your child's progress until he or she goes to school. You may also welcome the advice of a social worker if you have financial problems or are a single parent. Social workers can also help to arrange a home help if necessary.

Post-natal Check

If you had a difficult birth, you will probably have your six-week check-up back at the hospital. Write down all your questions before you go, as this is another good opportunity to find out 'why me?', and what methods of delivery to expect in your next pregnancy. You may have an X-ray of your pelvis taken so that its size and shape can be seen by the doctor and the possibility of a vaginal delivery considered for next time. If you are very small, then a repeat Caesarean will be necessary and this can be planned in advance.

Future Pregnancies

After a Caesarean birth you would be wise to wait at least a year before becoming pregnant again, so as not to stretch the scar tissue too soon.

Future Deliveries

If you have a small pelvis you will need to have all your babies delivered by Caesarean: how many can you have? Most doctors would recommend that you stop at three, providing the babies are all healthy. If you are very keen you can have more babies, although there is a greater risk of the scar tissue giving way in late pregnancy, and the operation itself can become technically more difficult after many Caesareans. Some doctors will sterilize you at the same time as a third Caesarean but others would prefer to wait for six weeks to three months (see Page 87).

If your pelvis is a good size and shape, you will be able to go into labour next time and may well have a normal delivery. The labour will be watched carefully to make sure the progress is normal and thus the previous scar is not stressed unduly (see Page 40). Once you have had a Caesarean, a home birth would be most unwise.

7 Personal Experiences

Three very different Caesarean Births

When pregnant for the first time, nine years ago, the one thing I didn't want at all costs was a Caesarean section, having seen patients of my medical student husband looking ill and in pain while other new mothers bustled about the ward chatting. However, as the time drew nearer I thought no more about it and was dismayed when, after my waters had broken two days previously, the cervix had not opened and I was told I would need a Caesarean. The surgeon warned me that it would be painful and uncomfortable but that the one thing that would make it worthwhile would be the baby in the cot beside me.

That made sense, and anyway I thought it would be a relief to have the baby. However, I had never had an operation before and found the mask unbearable and the whole paraphernalia disturbing. Instead of a husband beside me, participating in the amazing experience of the birth of our first baby, I was alone among alien cloaked and masked figures.

The next thing I was aware of was a voice saying that I was to be thrown away and I felt myself to be small and, to all intents and purposes, dead, lying at the bottom of a dustbin. I looked up towards the light in time to see my husband putting the lid on the bin, but I could not make him see or hear that I was still alive. Leering faces came and went; the horror of those hallucinations experienced on regaining consciousness remained with me up to the birth of my second child, causing a certain amount of dread of further anaesthesia.

Someone told me I had a boy but I didn't see my baby for three days so I had none of the satisfaction of him lying beside me as promised by the surgeon. The pain was intense and my inability to move, apart from the excruciating effort of hoisting myself up by the bars of the bed head, was distressing, as was the constant need to lie on my back. The nights were especially bad; from being healthy, happy and excited after an uneventful and joyful pregnancy, I felt I had been reduced to a feeble invalid.

The baby, when he was eventually brought to me, seemed something alien and detached; he seemed not to be mine because I had not experienced his birth. In spite of the late start, I did feed Sam myself, although resting the baby on a tender stomach was sometimes excruciating. Recovery seemed much slower than that of my neighbours and even now when I hear others talk of the wonder of birth, I feel a sense of loss, an incompleteness that I was incapable of having a baby normally and could share none of the experiences of labour and birth with those around me.

My stomach was tender for some time and the operation left me prone to cystitis. I think, too, that a Caesarean is extra worry for the father, who can have no share in the birth. It also limits, to a certain extent, the number of births a mother can expect.

My second experience of a Caesarean beat the planned 'Elective Caesarean' by one day. Because of my worry that hallucinations might recur, I was offered an epidural instead of general anaesthetic. This I accepted only to retract after fellow patients persuaded me that it would be awful to be awake during an operation and to see what was happening, all of which I believed, stupidly, having never met anyone who had had a Caesarean by epidural. I was given a drug to bring me quickly back to consciousness so I avoided the hallucinations, only to suffer an ileus (failure of the bowel to work properly) on the third day after the operation. I also learnt that there had been problems during the anaesthetic and the doctors had had to operate very quickly to save Jessica.

I remember the horror of waking the first morning to find a dressing revealing a vertical wound that I felt would never allow me to wear a bikini again. Not only was it a long, vertical scar, but because Jessica had to be got out quickly and because of the ileus that followed, it was puckered, red and swollen. It was embarrassing and ugly whereas the previous one had been low and horizontal with just a small drainage dent. Even now, I hate to see my stomach in the mirror, crisscrossed with lines.

When I was taken to see my baby the day after the birth, I could not imagine that she was mine—flabby, tube fed and dopey from the anaesthetic. The next few days I spent flat on my back after the ileus with tubes protruding from every orifice, only able to suck an ice cube and again with no baby in sight. After four days of this, I insisted on having my baby so that I could try, despite the tubes, to feed her. Gradually our relationship developed after its precarious start and I feel that, had she been my first baby, I would not have had the confidence to insist on her presence with me, and thus would never have successfully fed her or established any early contact with her.

After a second Caesarean I was even more protective of my scars, with an energetic two-year-old clambering over me at every opportunity. Everything physical suffered for some time, whether it was sexual relations, exercise or the day-to-day running of a home and family. With determination I managed and I don't remember ever being really depressed, but it was hard going.

In a vague attempt to exorcise the bad experience of earlier births, I longed for another child, determined this time to be in control, and to have as near natural a birth as I could. With the confidence of two previous Caesareans behind me and a greater knowledge of hospitals, I asked for a Caesarean by epidural. My husband was able to be with me so at last we could share the birth of our miracle baby. It was strange lying on the table knowing I was being cut open, yet feeling only a pulling and pushing, no pain. I asked my husband when the operation would start, only to be told that he could already see the baby's head! The birth itself took only minutes although the anaesthetic took a long time to administer but was far less frightening than a general, as I felt I could remain in control of what was happening and could at last participate in the birth. The moments I treasure are the ones of actually hearing my baby's first cry, hearing the words "it's a girl!" and holding her against my skin, covered as she was in blood and liquor, instead of being presented with a baby that was cleaned, polished and de-personalised in an incubator or cot as on previous occasions.

My feelings about her were incredible and still are, three years later, having seen her the moment she saw the world and having shared her birth with a loving and much-loved husband. She was always with me from then on. Neither of us had suffered the debilitating effects of the anaesthetic, so we enjoyed each other from the beginning. The pain, however, was even more excruciating once the epidural had worn off, perhaps because I had been sterilized at the same time. Nights especially were traumatic as I lay wondering if I dared to call a nurse yet again, or even if I could hoist myself up enough to reach the bell. In time the pain lessened, although I still suffered problems at home, with an infection in the tubes making housework and care of three children very difficult. Having Emily with me made up for everything—as my first surgeon had promised six years before!

This third birth also meant that my much resented scar could be excised and tidied up so that I feel happier in my bikini! A year after this birth I did have the scar injected by a plastic surgeon as it was still very pink and itchy. Now it is almost presentable and my only surviving problem is in telling my three beautiful children about the process of birth. "This is how a baby is born, BUT you came out a different way"!

Two Caesarean Births

When I was told that my first baby would need to be delivered by Caesarean (because of placenta praevia), my main feelings were of excitement and relief. Excitement because the nine long months of waiting and the *very* long last few days in the antenatal ward would be ended, no matter how abruptly. Relief because, ever since the moment when my GP had shaken his head over the baby's transverse position and decided to send me into hospital for checks, my husband and I had been suffering acute anxiety, the thought of malformation or still-birth very present in our minds (we had already had one late miscarriage). At last now something would actually happen and we would know the worst, or best. In fact the method of delivery seemed completely unimportant, compared to our worry as to whether the baby would be all right.

I was not unduly anxious about the operation itself, probably no more anxious than any first-time mother about the unknown experience of labour. However, it was irritating to be told by other expectant mums that I would be having a baby the easy way: just going to sleep and waking up to find the baby born, without any effort. I knew that there would be pain afterwards, even if I missed out on labour pains!

It is indescribably strange to go to sleep as one person and be woken an instant later (as it seems) as two people. Completely befuddled by anaesthetic, I was just able to understand that we had a daughter. She had breathing problems and was rushed to the Special Care Baby Unit. My husband saw her for a moment, but I don't remember doing so. Twenty-four hours later I was taken to the SCBU and, again, it was rather like a strange dream, to be taken into a room full of babies, and to look at them all, wondering which one was mine. I think I felt like an adoptive mother, being introduced to her future child. It was hard to believe she had been born from my body. However, we were lucky in that my husband and I could visit the SCBU any time, hold our baby's hand, touch her, cuddle her for a short time, and I was helped to breast-feed her. These early contacts were vital to dispel that first feeling of unreality and detachment, to bring home the fact that this was truly our baby.

Personal Experiences

For my son's birth I requested an epidural anaesthetic. Beforehand there were the same feelings of excitement, but a great deal more apprehension (I am very squeamish). My NCT relaxation exercises helped greatly, and I felt I was playing some sort of participatory role. Amazingly quickly, perhaps after ten minutes, the surgeon announced "it's a boy!" and handed me the baby. My feelings of joy and fulfilment were more intense than any I have ever experienced before or since; for two or three days I was on a wonderful "high", quite drunk with delight in this new baby. I tried to put him to the breast while on the operating table, pretty awkward while lying flat and hitched up to drips, but we managed something. This time there was no Special Care, no muzziness or sickness from the anaesthetic. As soon as I was sewn up, we were simply taken to the post-natal ward, as if it had been a normal delivery, feeling happy and astonishingly well.

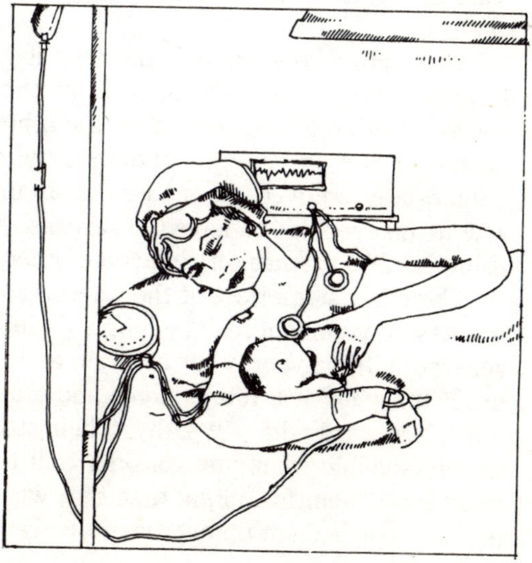

It is perfectly possible to feed and cuddle the baby while the operation is still going on and you are being stitched up

The one person who really missed out was my husband, who very much wanted to be present at the birth of his children. Missing this experience has been a great sadness for him, although I don't think it has affected his very loving relationship with both of them. I must add that the hospital does allow fathers to be present at Caesarean births, although very few avail themselves of the privilege. I think, if our positions had been reversed, I would not have been able to watch him being cut up either.

I found no problems in breast-feeding my babies, given some pillows and some help lifting them to the breast at first. It is very frustrating though, to be unable to pick up your baby when you wish, without having to ring for a nurse. For the first couple of days after the operation I certainly felt convinced that I would split open if I made any sudden movements (I was terrified of sneezing!) and it was impossible to bend over to pick up the baby from its cot. The nurses were very busy, and I was dependent on the other mothers in the ward and grateful to them for giving me my baby when he cried.

That period soon passed, and then it was just the same hospital routine as for all the other mothers, but for longer of course. The great ordeal (and all the other Caesarean patients I have ever met agree on this point) is the dreadful day when the stitches are removed. I am sure that if any of the surgeons who sew us up ever had to have Caesareans, they might consider using soluble stitches, or find some other solution.

The other side effect of the Caesarean operation is the toll it takes on your family. The long stay in hospital involves long separation from your other children and this I think causes problems when you return home and must influence their attitude towards the new baby. Their attitude is very understandable when you consider that their mother is not only away from them for a long time but, when she returns, is unable to pick them up and has to be careful about many activities for the first three months at home. But these are minor problems. My two Caesarean operations have given me two beautiful, healthy children and really nothing else matters.

A Breech Birth

The birth of my second baby could easily have been by Caesarean as she was a breech delivery. It was a bit of a shock to be told the baby was in a breech position. I'd had a normal, straightforward pregnancy until 37 weeks when I thought the whole of my insides were rotating as my baby turned into this abnormal position. Whatever the reason, there was little space for her to turn back and there she remained until her birth three weeks later. It was strange to feel this obvious little head bobbing about where the kicking should be—I almost felt I could communicate verbally with this little creature.

My own doctor diagnosed a breech position, confirmed by a senior partner who also attempted to turn her externally. It was very uncomfortable as she was reluctant to be moved, so he decided to leave well alone and I was sent to see the Consultant. Fortunately he is a great believer in vaginal breech delivery wherever possible and an X-ray confirmed that my pelvis was big enough.

I needed to be mentally prepared to approach the birth with confidence, and I consulted as many people as possible about likely difficulties of a breech delivery. Entering hospital at 40 weeks I was well informed, and aware of the possible complications.

My labour was started off with a pessary to soften the cervix and by mid-morning I was on my way. I had asked for an anaesthetist to be present, to keep my options open for an epidural, which many of the medical staff had advised for a breech delivery. I was very dubious about this sort of anaesthetic, knowing it would immobilise me and had associated risks, but I was prepared to accept it if labour was hard, and for the sake of the baby's safe arrival, as a slow, careful delivery of the head is essential when the head is delivered after the body. I was also informed that forceps would almost certainly be used.

Labour progressed very rapidly with irregular, close contractions, and I had an extremely strong urge to push at only 3-4cm dilation of the cervix. I was aware that this could be a problem, as the baby's bottom is smaller than the head and is pushed into the opening cervix. I decided to have an epidural to help stop me pushing and to relieve the pain in my back. I was grateful for the relief the epidural offered but I was surprised to find I still had an overwhelming urge to push. I had a four-hour labour with periods of shakiness, sweatiness and fatigue and I wished it was all over and everyone would go away so that I could sleep.

As the second stage of labour began I was aware that this birth was anything but normal as it was to be witnessed by six student midwives, an anaesthetist and an obstetrician were on standby in case of an emergency Caesarean and a paediatrician was there to examine the baby immediately. The epidural was topped up as forceps were going to be used, but I was still able to feel my baby travel through the birth canal. I was hoisted in stirrups and baby's bottom appeared followed without difficulty by the legs and body; to help her I had been given a rather large episiotomy. It was a very tense moment for us as she was held by her legs and the forceps inserted and her head very carefully delivered, a perfect shape without damage.

Looking back, it was an exciting experience, although not as fulfilling as the birth of my first child, which was managed without drugs or epidural. The epidural worried me, especially as it took several hours for the numbness to wear off, due to the last-minute topping up. I was happy to have experienced the birth without the necessity of a Caesarean. My recovery was that of a normal birth with a little extra bruising from the forceps and episiotomy.

Some other quotes

On learning that a Caesarean Birth would be necessary:

"I was very upset because I wanted a normal birth. A Caesarean seemed too clinical, no mad dash in the middle of the night, no timing of contractions, is it—isn't it? However, once I had come to terms with the decision I made the best use of the days left and booked to have my hair done and had a night out with my husband the day before I had to go into hospital."

"I was totally unprepared and so the thought of going into an operating theatre filled me with horror. I was bitterly disappointed that I would not be able to deliver the baby myself."

"At 9.30 on Saturday morning I was told an emergency Caesarean would be necessary because the baby was distressed. I burst into tears—all those hours in labour."

During a Caesarean under epidural anaesthetic:

"In the end it was a marvellous experience: every care was taken setting up the epidural with explanations all the way, and I felt the anaesthetist was my true friend and ally. My husband was present and held my hands throughout. As Sarah was born I felt the sensations but not the pain and I saw Sarah immediately. There wasn't any sickness and I was conscious and alert all day until the evening sleep."

After a Caesarean Birth:

"I rather resented the baby and blamed him. I did feel cheated, as though I had been given a baby that could have been anyone's. I missed the actual first sight of the baby, knowing it was mine, the sense of relief and achievement and also my husband's company and pleasure. He found my having the operation a great strain, and not an experience he would like to repeat."

"There was quite a bit of pain to begin with but the hospital was very good and would give me painkillers when required."

"I couldn't move, it was too painful: I couldn't even reach the water. I called out but only a whisper came so no-one heard."

"Apart from an internal infection which I had for six weeks after the birth, I did get gradually back to normal, although for some weeks any clothing against the scar was very uncomfortable."

"I was very tired and felt poorly for a long time; the baby was unsettled for months. However, as time went on Andrew was much improved, and by 18 months I was much better and Andrew turned into a delightful boy."

"Baby Tom is 2½ years old and worth every minute of his difficult birth—more-or-less!"

Last Words

Between 1958 and 1970, the percentage of babies delivered by Caesarean almost doubled, from 2.7 to 4.5%, and from 1970 to 1978 the rate almost doubled again, to 8.7%. In some hospitals the proportion of women delivered by forceps may be as low as one in fifty, whereas in others it is as high as one in five. As nutrition has improved over the last 25 years and younger people are taller than their parents, one might have expected the rate of difficult delivery to fall rather than rise, but babies also tend to be bigger.

Nobody wants to return to the days when women laboured for days and an exhausted mother gave birth to a dead or handicapped baby, but as Caesareans have become safer, some doctors feel they are sometimes used too freely. If labour is induced before the woman is ready to deliver, it may fail and so a Caesarean is done; thus, very critical review of the indications for induction and the chance of it being successful will, it is hoped, reduce the number of Caesarean sections performed today. Monitoring the baby's heartbeat and testing the acidity of the baby's blood (see Page 24) together form a reliable method of detecting a baby in distress during labour, whereas monitoring the baby's heartbeat alone can be misleading and has been shown to increase the Caesarean section rate, without necessarily saving more babies. Some of the rise is explained by the ability of paediatricians to save very small babies; in the past most of these babies were unlikely to survive and therefore operating on the mother was not considered justifiable.

Pregnant women want to trust their obstetricians, and not to fight the medical profession, but doctors can hold very different views about the way to manage labour and delivery, and it is worth talking to your own GP about the policies of your local consultants. If you can't stand the idea of a long labour, and would like an epidural for pain relief, and to have your baby's heartbeat monitored continuously, then Consultant A may be the right person for you. If you want to start labour naturally, have no drugs and deliver in the squatting position, preferably without an episiotomy, then Consultant B may share your views.

Fortunately, in this country doctors do not perform operations because of the fees they will receive, and obstetricians are trained to do their best to assist women to have a healthy baby; so, once in labour, trust your doctor's judgement—he will be doing what is believed to be the best for both of you.

Useful Addresses and Further Reading

Useful Addresses

La Leche League of Great Britain, B.M. 3424, London WC1 6XX. Tel: 01-404 5011.
National Childbirth Trust, 9 Queensborough Terrace, London W2 3TB. Tel: 01-229 9319/9310.
Caesarean Support Group of Cambridge. Ann Watson, 7 Green Street, Willingham, Cambridgeshire.
AIMS (The Association for Improvements in Maternity Services). Elizabeth Cockerell, 21 Franklin Road, Hitchin, Hertfordshire SG4 0NE. Tel: 0462 2179.
Maternity Alliance, 309 Kentish Town Road, London NW5. Tel: 01-267 7477.
The Twins Clubs Association. Margaret Cann, Roma, Grange Road, Ash, Aldershot, Hampshire. Tel: 0252 310611.
Family Planning Information Service. Margaret Pyke House, 27/35 Mortimer Street, London W1A 4QW. Tel: 01-580 9360.
Mind (National Association for Mental Health), 22 Harley Street, London W1N 2ED. Tel: 01-637 0741.
The National Stillbirth Study Group, 66 Harley Street, London W1N 1AE.
Health Education Council, 78 New Oxford Street, London WC1A 1AH.

Further Reading

The Caesarean Birth Experience	B. Donovan, Beacon Press, 1978
The Experience of Childbirth	S. Kitzinger, Penguin, 1982
The Good Birth Guide	S. Kitzinger, Fontana, 1979
Pregnancy Questions Answered	G. Chamberlain, Churchill Livingstone, 1982
A Child is Born	L. Nilsson, Faber & Faber, 1981
Talking with Mothers	D. Breen, Jill Norman, 1981
The Experience of Breastfeeding	S. Kitzinger, Penguin, 1979
Breast-feeding after a Caesarean Birth	La Leche League International, Information Sheet No. 80
Nourishing Your Unborn Child	P. S. Williams, Avon Books, 1974
Essential Exercises in the Child-Bearing Year	Elizabeth Noble, Houghton & Miflin, 1976
Depression after Childbirth	K. Dalton, OUP, 1980
Our Bodies, Our Selves	A. Phillips and J. Rakausen, Penguin, 1978
The Womanly Art of Breast-Feeding	La Leche League International, 1981
A Mother's guide to breast-feeding and mothering the premature or hospitalized sick infant	La Leche League International, Information Sheet No. 109
New Life Book of Exercises for Childbirth	A. & J. Balaskas, Sidgwick & Jackson, 1979
The First Relationship: Infant and Mother	D. Stern, 1977
The Good Health Guide for Women	C. Cooke and S. Dorkin, revised British Edition, J. Turner & W. Savage, Hamlyn, 1981
The Birth Control Book	H. Shapiro, Penguin, 1980.
The British Way of Birth	E. Rantzen and G. Bourne, Pan, 1982
You after childbirth	J. McKenna, M. Polden and M. Williams. A Churchill Livingstone Patient Handbook
Twins	C. Zentner, Macdonald, Edinburgh, 1984

Susan Michelle Moll

Wege der Bewusstwerdung

http://www.susan-moll.com

Danksagung
Ich danke Dir lieber Christus, dass Du mich inspiriert hast dieses Buch zu schreiben und mich ständig unterstützt hast.

Danke lieber Peter, dass Du mich immer wieder angefeuert hast weiterzumachen, und das Buch zu vollenden, ohne Deine Hilfe hätte ich es nicht geschafft.

Danke liebe Martina für Deine wunderbare Übersetzung und Zusammenarbeit.

ISBN 3-8334-2011-1

http://www.susan-moll.com
E-Mail: islandoflight@susan-moll.com
Herstellung und Verlag:
Books on Demand GmbH, Norderstedt
http://www.bod.de

Autorin: Susan Michelle Moll
Cover & Rückseite: Silvia Summer, Maui - Hawaii
Nachwort: Seite 122 und Gebet der Vollkommenheit: Seite 124 durch Mirra Rose
Übersetzung: Martina Hochmair, Wallern
Satz und Layout: Peter Polz, Stainz

Inhaltsverzeichnis

Vorwort

Dieses Buch wurde von den Meistern des Lichts zum Zwecke der mühelosen Erlangung des Christusbewusstseins entworfen. Freut Euch, meine Geliebten, denn Ihr werdet wieder in Harmonie, Fülle, Frieden und Freude leben können, wie es für diesen wunderschönen Planeten Erde schon seit jeher vorgesehen war! Bleibt noch wenig länger standhaft, und die Belohnungen werden über Euer menschliches Verständnis hinausreichen. Auf der Erde und in der gesamten Menschheit werden wieder Friede und Liebe vorherrschen.

Stellt Euch vor, wie das sein wird! Nehmt Euch wirklich einen Augenblick lang Zeit – und denkt darüber nach, was Ihr an dem, das gegenwärtig auf dem Planeten geschieht, alles verändern würdet. Macht Euch im Geiste davon Notizen oder, noch besser, erstellt eine Liste von allem, das Ihr transformieren würdet. Meditiert jeden Tag darüber und bedankt Euch dafür herzlich beim Schöpfer.

In der Zukunft der Erde wird sich eine gewaltige Wende vollziehen. Übernehmt die Verantwortung dafür, dass Ihr die Mitschöpfer seid, welche Ihr verkörpert und manifestiert viele wunderbare Dinge, nach denen sich Eure Herzen und Euer Geist sehnen. Meine Geliebten, es ist für jeden Einzelnen von Euch Zeit, aktiv zu werden. Die Zeit der Untätigkeit ist vorüber. Marschiert voran, jeder Einzelne meiner geliebten Krieger, nehmt Eure Macht wieder in Anspruch und werdet zu den Meistern, die Ihr in Wirklichkeit seid!

Vorstellung der Autorin

Susan Michelle Moll, die Verfasserin dieses Buches, ist die Mutter von drei Kindern: Alexander Richard, geboren 1978, Melanie Natascha, geboren 1981, und Serena Louise Moll, geboren 1986. Alle drei Kinder leben gegenwärtig mit ihren Eltern in Maui, Hawaii. Zuvor hatte die Familie zweiundzwanzig Jahre lang in Bayern, Deutschland, gelebt.

Sue hat den Großteil ihres Lebens dafür gewidmet, anderen zu dienen, ihre Kinder großzuziehen und im Familienbetrieb mitzuhelfen. Sie ist eine ausgebildete Aura-Soma-Farbtherapeutin und hat nun Freude daran, ihre Sitzungen mit den heilenden Schwingungen der wertvollen BioGenesis-Instrumente mit anderen teilen zu können. Diese Instrumente können Gleichgewicht und Harmonie erzeugen, Gesundheit und Vitalität wiederherstellen und die Lebensziele manifestieren. Die BioGenesis-Instrumente sind stets erneuernd, stets erfrischend und stets wiederherstellend. Diese Technologie wurde aus den Zeiten von Atlantis überliefert. Vor zehntausenden Jahren funktionierte diese Technologie auf Erden. Die Erde und die Menschheit freuen sich über die Rückkehr des Lichts von BioGenesis. Sue hat das Gefühl, dass sie jahrelang geduldig auf die Rückkehr dieser Heilungsinstrumente gewartet hat, und ist sehr dankbar und glücklich, dass sie Cindy und Terry Johnson und ihren Instrumenten im August 2000 auf Maui vorgestellt wurde. Ich danke Gott für den göttlichen Zeitplan und die Verbindungen!

Sie verfügt außerdem über die Fähigkeit, mit ihrem höheren Selbst, den höheren Reichen, den aufgestiegenen Meistern und Engeln zu kommunizieren, und beschreibt Sie im Buch als »Spirit«. Sie schreibt bereits seit mehreren Jahren persönliche Botschaften nieder und fühlt sich nun zuversichtlich genug, andere an dem teilhaben zu lassen, was ihr aufgrund ihrer eigenen Erfahrung als „Wahrheit“ bekannt ist.

Sue und ihre Familie wurden 1996 dazu angeleitet, ihr Unternehmen in Herrsching, Bayern, zu verkaufen und nach Maui zu übersiedeln, ohne dabei zu wissen, was die Zukunft mit sich bringen würde. Sue hat die letzten Jahre damit verbracht, alte Muster zu erkennen, zu akzeptieren und loszulassen. Und auch damit, ihre Macht jeden Tag etwas mehr zu beanspruchen und Augenblick für Augenblick der Führung von Spirit zu folgen. Sie hat gelernt, im Jetzt zu leben und dabei alles, was ist, zu akzeptieren. Einige Jahre zuvor hatte sie in ihrem florierenden Tenniszentrum in Bayern eine Insel des Lichts (= ein kleines Heilungszentrum) gegründet. Hier wurden die Aura-Soma-Flaschen im Empfangsbereich ausgestellt, damit sie von allen bewundert werden konnten. Die Insel des Lichts diente dazu, die Heilung auf viele verschiedene Arten voranzubringen.

Nur durch ihr Vertrauen in ihre Führung und indem sie ihrem Herzen folgte, hat sie den Punkt erreicht, an dem sie heute steht. Stets voller Vertrauen, stets geführt und stets von Augenblick zu Augenblick lebend, in Erwartung des nächsten Wunders, das Spirit bewirken wird. Stets voller Dankbarkeit für alles, was Gott ihr und ihrer Familie gegeben hat, das wunderschöne Haus, in dem sie leben, und vor allem voller Dankbarkeit dafür, dass sie die Möglichkeit hat, dem Schöpfer auf der wunderschönen Insel Maui zu dienen.

Bevor wir mit diesem kleinen Buch fortfahren, würde Sue gerne schildern, wie sie diese Informationen empfangen hat, und auch ein wenig über ihren Weg und die Schwierigkeiten, die sie zu bewältigen hatte, erzählen:

Obwohl ich schon länger meditiert und die Botschaften, die ich empfing, niedergeschrieben hatte, bereitete es mir stets große Schwierigkeiten, zu mir selbst und den Informationen, die ich empfing, Vertrauen zu haben. Es war ein sehr langsamer Prozess, der einige Jahre dauerte. Bis vor ein paar Monaten sträubte ich mich dagegen, diese Botschaften mit meiner Familie und meinen

Freunden zu teilen. Ich hatte Angst vor der damit verbundenen Verantwortung. Nun ist mir klar, dass jeder für sich selbst verantwortlich ist. Jeder Mensch muss für sich herausfinden, ob die Informationen für ihn der Wahrheit entsprechen. Ich kann nur das, was ich empfange und für meine Wahrheit halte, weitergeben, und es ist die Angelegenheit jedes Einzelnen, der dieses Buch liest, herauszufinden, ob dies für ihn der Wahrheit entspricht oder nicht.

Erst jetzt, dank der Ermutigung durch meine Familie und meine Freunde, bin ich in der Lage, diese einfachen Informationen in großer Freude zu teilen, da ich weiß, dass sie für mich der Wahrheit entsprechen.

Dies ist etwas, das ich mit jeder Zelle meines Seins empfangen und erlebt habe. Ich glaube, die Meister wussten, dass dies die einzige Möglichkeit war, wie sie mich dazu bewegen konnten, die Informationen hervorzubringen – indem ich mich selbst erlebte und wusste, dass dies die Wahrheit war! Ich danke ihnen von Herzen dafür, dass sie so viel Geduld mit mir hatten. Ich bin nun bereit, und das Schreiben bereitet mir so viel Freude und Aufregung! Der innerste Kern meines Wesens möchte sich selbst Ausdruck verleihen. Zum ersten Mal in meinem Leben habe ich das Gefühl, dass ich wirklich am Leben bin und dass ich eine Aufgabe habe. Ich bin ewig dankbar dafür. Jedes

Mal habe ich eine neue Erkenntnis, und dies ist eine aufregende und ermächtigende Sache.

Ich habe viele dunkle Zeiten durchgemacht und bin mit der Tiefe der Verzweiflung in Berührung gekommen. Während einer Meditation erkannte ich eines Tages, dass das Ego wie ‚der Teufel in mir' war, der versuchte, mich zu beherrschen und mich daran zu hindern, Erleuchtung zu erlangen. In dem Moment, an dem ich dies begriff, war ich entschlossen, nicht mehr zuzulassen, dass mein Ego die Oberhand über mich gewinnt! Manchmal verfalle ich noch in selbst erschaffene Depression und Verzweiflung. Wenn ich es jedoch der mächtigen ICH-BIN-Gegenwart gestatte, das Kommando über meine menschliche Schöpfung zu übernehmen, bin ich mit Hilfe der in diesem Buch enthaltenen Schlüssel dazu fähig, aus dem Ganzen wieder herauszukommen.

Ich glaube, dass dieses Leben eine kontinuierliche Reise ist – manchmal erklimmen wir die Höhen und sehen das Licht, sind entzückt und erfüllt von Freude, Dankbarkeit und Glückseligkeit, aber dann fallen wir wieder hinunter in das nächste Tal, um neue Lektionen zu lernen, die wir zu meistern haben. Obwohl ich mir selbst auf jeder Ebene Leid verursacht habe, hat sich dies aufgrund der Lektionen, die ich daraus gelernt habe, gelohnt. Ich bete dafür, dass die Menschen einen einfacheren Weg finden werden, durch die dunkle Nacht der Seele hindurchzugehen. Ich weiß, dass jeder Mensch, der sich dafür entscheidet, diese Reise anzutreten, dazu beitragen wird, dass es für diejenigen, die nachkommen, leichter sein wird.

Bei den wichtigsten Lektionen, die ich erteilt bekam, ging es darum, dass ich lernen sollte, mich selbst ungeachtet all meiner menschlichen Fehler zu lieben und mir zu vergeben. Ich habe gelernt, mich selbst zu akzeptieren, wie ich bin, ohne dabei perfekt sein zu müssen. Mittlerweile bin ich so weit, dass ich Vertrauen in mich selbst und meine Fähigkeiten habe.

Ich verbrachte den Großteil meines Lebens damit, das zu tun, was alle anderen von mir wollten. Jeder Augenblick wurde von dem Wunsch, andere Leute zufrieden stellen zu wollen, angeregt.

„Nachdem ich tief in mein Inneres eingetaucht war, habe ich herausgefunden, wer ich in Wirklichkeit bin und warum ich hier bin. Ich verstehe jeden Tag besser, dass es vollkommen an mir selbst liegt, mein Leben so zu gestalten, wie ich es haben möchte. Wenn ich mich auf Dankbarkeit, Liebe, Anerkennung und das Annehmen von allem, was existiert, konzentriere, fließen die Tage in großer Freude und Glückseligkeit dahin. Wenn ich mich auf die Dinge konzentriere, an denen es mir fehlt, raten Sie mal, wovon ich dann mehr bekomme?

Die ersten eineinhalb Jahre auf Maui verbrachte ich damit, mich selbst zu heilen. Jeden Tag fragte ich Spirit, was ich heute tun sollte, und dann folgte die Antwort: ‚Sei einfach!' Ich ging an den Strand, um zu schwimmen und stellte fest, dass neben mir im Wasser ständig Bienen schwammen! Es ist stets sehr amüsant zu erfahren, dass Spirit so einen wundervollen Sinn für Humor hat. Dies fiel mir sehr schwer, da ich stets eine ‚Tuende' gewesen war. Ich hatte jegliche erdenkliche Art von Angst durchgemacht: Angst, nicht würdig zu sein, weil ich überhaupt nichts tat; Angst, dass uns das Geld ausgehen würde; Angst, dass man unser Visum nicht verlängern würde; Angst, dass ich meine Mission verfehlt hatte; Angst, dass ich mich vielleicht vergeblich bemüht hatte; Angst, dass ich vollkommen aus einer ‚normalen' Gesellschaft ausgestiegen sei (ich hatte aufgehört, als Reaktion darauf, was die Leute dachten, zu leben).

Und dann erkannte ich eines Tages, dass ich Geld mit Macht und Erfolg mit Karriere gleichgesetzt hatte. Es kam mir so vor, als wäre ich ein Niemand, wenn ich keines dieser Dinge (Geld oder Karriere) hatte! Mein unbewusster Verstand wusste natürlich, dass das nicht stimmte, aber die Enthüllung dieses subtilen Glaubenssatzes war der Anfang für die Befreiung von einer Begrenzung dieser Art.

„An diesem Punkt fand ich meine Freiheit oder wenigstens einen Teil davon. Ich begann zu akzeptieren, dass ich hier war, um mich selbst von all diesen alten

Mustern zu heilen. Ich konnte sehr dankbar dafür sein, dass ich zu dieser Zeit in einer Position war, in der ich nicht jeden Tag zur Arbeit gehen musste. Ich konnte mir aussuchen, wie ich meine Zeit gestalten wollte. Ich konnte an den Strand gehen, schwimmen, das Tanzbein schwingen, lesen, schreiben, auf Seide malen, spazieren gehen, einkaufen gehen. Ich konnte es mir selbst gestatten, das zu tun, wonach auch immer mein Herz verlangte. Wie gesegnet ich doch war!

Anstatt mich auf all das zu konzentrieren, was ich nicht tat, begann ich, meine Aufmerksamkeit auf die wunderbare Gelegenheit zu richten, die mir geboten wurde. Sobald ich dies als meinen Weg akzeptiert hatte, begann ich zu entdecken, was ich tun sollte. Von diesem Tag an empfand ich viel Freude, Glückseligkeit, Anerkennung und Liebe für alles, was in meinem Leben existierte. Ich bin wirklich dankbar für alles, was mir mein Leben dargeboten hat, und möchte meinen Dank dafür zum Ausdruck bringen.

Ich weiß nun, dass ein Teil meiner Mission darin besteht, dieses Buch zu schreiben und die darin enthaltenen Schlüssel zu lehren. Als Erstes musste ich lernen, jede Situation in meinem Leben als vollkommen hinzunehmen, und dann konnte der ‚Zauber' beginnen.

Im Juni 1998 wurde ich gefragt, ob ich bereit sei, mir dieses kleine Buch, das der Meister Jesus Christus verfassen wollte, diktieren zu lassen. Es sollte in einer deutlichen und einfachen Sprache geschrieben sein, sodass es jeder Mann, jede Frau und jedes Kind verstehen könnte.

Ich war einverstanden. Und so nahm es seinen Anfang, indem ich nach meiner morgendlichen Meditation an den meisten Tagen Informationen empfing. Erstaunlicherweise war die Wahl des Zeitpunkts immer perfekt, und die durchgegebenen Informationen passten perfekt zu dem, was ich persönlich durchmachte. Ich habe tatsächlich jeden einzelnen der Prozesse in diesem Buch in die Praxis umgesetzt. Oft verspürte ich einen großen Widerstand gegen die dargebrachten Wahrheiten. Es gelang mir, zahlreiche alte Glaubenssysteme und Muster aufzulösen. Allerdings war dies nicht immer eine einfache oder angenehme Erfahrung. Sich die Wahrheit über mich selbst anzusehen und meine Fehler einzugestehen, ist keine Sache, die ich als angenehm empfinde. Allerdings überwiegt die Ermächtigung, die mit der Anerkennung der Wahrheit einhergeht, bei weitem gegenüber den Seitenhieben, die dem Ego dabei versetzt werden.

Ich habe intensiv mit der mächtigen violetten Flamme und dem weißgoldenen Lichtstrahl gearbeitet. Ich habe täglich meine mächtige ICH-BIN-Gegenwart um Unterstützung angerufen, und das Gesetz der Vergebung angeordnet und angerufen. Von allen Instrumenten, die ich im Laufe der letzten zwölf Jahre verwendet habe, waren diese hier am hilfreichsten. Diese Übungen mache ich natürlich zusätzlich zu meiner täglichen Meditation. Dies hat mich in meinem Herzen beruhigt und zentriert und mich an einen Ort geführt, an dem vollkommener Friede, Liebe und Freude herrschen.

Ich gebe jedem von Ihnen den Rat, den Tag mit einem Gebet und einer Meditation zu beginnen. Ich habe den Eindruck, dass mein Tag voller Leichtigkeit und Anmut dahinfließt, wenn ich das tue. Verbinden Sie diese Instrumente mit den in diesem Buch enthaltenen Schlüsseln, und ich versichere Ihnen, dass Ihr Leben eine gewaltige Wendung in eine äußerst positive Richtung nehmen wird!

Für den Fall, dass jemand von Ihnen die Bücher erwerben möchte, die mir am meisten geholfen haben, habe ich sie nachstehend aufgelistet:

The „I AM" Discourses (Anm. d. Ü.: auf Deutsch nicht erhältlich, Titel in etwa: Die „ICH-BIN"-Diskurse) vom aufgestiegenen Meister Saint Germain, durchgegeben von Godfrey Ray King, St. Germain Press Inc., 1120 Stonehedge Drive, Schaumburg, Illinois 60194. Es gibt zwölf unterschiedliche Bände, und ich würde Ihnen empfehlen, mit Band I, Unveiled Mysteries (= Enträtselte Geheimnisse) zu beginnen.

„Chakren – die sieben Zentren von Kraft und Heilung" von Dr. Caroline Myss, Droemer Knaur Verlag, „Auf Schwingen des Lichts . . . Erzengel Michael spricht" von Ronna Herman, Ventla Verlag

Sämtliche „Kryon"-Bücher, die von Lee Carroll verfasst wurden.

Bei sämtlichen Informationen, die ich mit Ihnen teile, bitte ich Sie, von Ihrem eigenen Urteilsvermögen Gebrauch zu machen. Nehmen Sie sich das heraus, was sich für Sie richtig anfühlt, wenden Sie es an und heben Sie den Rest für eine Verwendung zu einem späteren Zeitpunkt auf!

Lassen Sie zu, dass diese Botschaften Ihr Herz und Ihre Seele ansprechen werden. Lassen Sie dann Ihr Herz und Ihre Seele entscheiden, ob sich diese Informationen für Sie wahr anhören. Ich hoffe aufrichtig, dass ein Teil dieser Informationen Ihnen und Ihren Familien helfen wird. Diese einfachen Wahrheiten können Ihr Leben verbessern, wenn Sie zulassen, dass der Prozess beginnt. Jeder Mensch wird in seinem Leben und seiner Welt Veränderungen gegenüberstehen, da in den kommenden Zeiten nur die Wahrheit bestehen bleiben wird.

Ich halte Kurse zu den in diesem Buch enthaltenen Informationen und bringe den Leuten Möglichkeiten bei, diese Schlüssel in unserem täglichen Leben anzuwenden.

Für nähere Informationen schreiben Sie bitte an:
islandoflight@susan-moll.com

Danksagungen

Ich danke der mächtigen ICH-BIN-Gegenwart, Christus, Saint Germain, Mutter Maria und all den Meistern des Lichts ewig dafür, dass sie mir in dieser sehr herausfordernden Zeit meines Lebens beigestanden haben. Ich möchte mich auch bei Harry, meinem Ehemann, und bei meinen drei Kindern bedanken für ihre unaufhörliche Liebe und Unterstützung während den schwierigen Zeiten.

Ich möchte auch meinen wunderbaren Eltern für ihre unablässige Liebe und Unterstützung danken. Sie waren mit vielen Ängsten konfrontiert, als meine Familie jegliche offenbare Sicherheit zurückließ, um unserer Führung nach Hawaii zu folgen. Ich danke ihnen dafür, dass sie so verständnisvoll waren, uns immer geholfen haben und dass sie losgelassen und gestattet haben, dass wir von Gott geführt werden. Ich liebe und schätze sie beide und bin ewig dankbar für alles, was sie mir beigebracht haben!

Ich möchte auch meiner lieben Freundin Silvia, die das wunderschöne Cover entworfen und gemalt hat, Dank und Anerkennung aussprechen. Ihren großartigen Bildern ist es zu verdanken, dass dieses Buch ein ganz besonderes Bild und ein ganz besonderes Gefühl vermittelt. Ich danke ihr dafür, dass sie immer für mich da war, wenn ich einen Freund brauchte, und für all den Spaß, den wir gemeinsam haben, wenn wir das Tanzbein schwingen und am Strand spielen!

Weiters möchte ich mich bei meiner lieben Freundin Mirra, meiner Seelenschwester, für ihre unaufhörliche Unterstützung und Liebe bedanken. Sie zählt zu den besten Freunden, die ich habe, und sie hat mir so sehr geholfen. Ich danke ihr dafür, dass sich mich ermutigt hat, diese Arbeit zu tun, und dafür, dass sie mir auf so wundervolle Weise mein Spiegelbild ist.

Ich möchte auch Sahara, die dieses Buch für mich redigiert hat, meinen herzlichen Dank aussprechen. Ich bin sehr dankbar für ihre Geduld, Beratung und Erfahrung auf diesem Gebiet. Ich danke Dir so sehr, meine geliebte Schwester. Ohne Dich hätte ich dies nicht zustande gebracht!

Ich möchte mich auch bei meiner lieben Freundin Harriet bedanken, nicht nur dafür, dass sie eine wundervolle Freundin ist, sondern auch dafür, dass sie Pamela Curlee in mein Leben gebracht hat, die mir Cindy und Terry Johnson und die großartigen BioGenesis-Instrumente vorstellte. Von dem Moment, an dem ich Pam kennen lernte, tat mir mein Herz weh, es war eine deutliche Wiedererkennung aus der Vergangenheit, und wir stellten sofort auf allen Ebenen eine Verbindung zueinander her.

Ich danke Pam, Harriet, Cindy, Terry und natürlich auch dem geliebten aufgestiegenen Meister Lantos dafür, dass ich endlich die wertvollen BioGenesis-Instrumente gefunden habe, die mit Sicherheit einen Teil meiner Lebensarbeit darstellen, und dafür bin ich ewig dankbar. Ich danke Euch aus tiefstem Herzen für alles, was Ihr im Einzelnen dazu beigetragen habt, um den göttlichen Plan zu vervollkommnen.

Gott ist so gut, und er hat in jedem Augenblick alles perfekt arrangiert, obwohl wir manchmal nicht dieser Ansicht sind und ungeduldig werden! Und dabei gehört Geduld in diesem Leben zu meinen wichtigsten Lektionen! Ich möchte Euch allen nochmals herzlich danken.

Teil I

Kapitel eins

Die grundlegenden Schritte in Richtung Meisterschaft sind äußerst einfach und für jeden Einzelnen verfügbar, solange Sie bereit sind, den Blick nach innen zu richten und alles, was Sie finden, anzuerkennen und anzunehmen!

Wenn Sie die in diesem Buch enthaltenen Schritte und Schlüssel beachten, können Sie sicher sein, dass Sie zu jenem Meister werden, von dem Sie vergessen haben, dass Sie dieser Meister sind!

Schlüssel Nummer eins: Verantwortung

Die Verantwortung für Ihr eigenes Leben zu übernehmen, ist der Schlüssel Nummer eins. Alles, was Sie in Ihrem Leben erschaffen, unterliegt Ihrer Verantwortung. Akzeptieren Sie diese Wahrheit und seien Sie sich bewusst, dass Sie alles, was geschieht, allein erschaffen haben, vom Anfang bis zum Ende!

In jedem Augenblick wurde jeder Gedanke, jedes Wort und jede Tat von Ihnen selbst erschaffen. Wenn Sie Liebe aussenden – raten Sie mal, was dann zu Ihnen zurückkehren wird – Liebe. Wenn Sie Zorn, Angst oder Verzweiflung aussenden, wird auch dies wieder zu Ihnen zurückkehren, und so weiter.

Beobachten Sie in jedem Augenblick Ihre Gedanken, Worte und Taten. Wenn Sie liebevolle Gedanken hegen, wird die Liebe fortbestehen und sich ausdehnen. Wenn Sie lieblose Gedanken hegen, werden diese fortbestehen und sich ausdehnen. Dies ist jene Ursache und Wirkung, die uns von der Welt rund um uns widergespiegelt wird, da wir in jedem Augenblick Schöpfer sind. Vergessen Sie dies bitte niemals!

Erinnern Sie sich an das einfache „Gesetz der Einheit“ und daran, dass mit Ihrer Hilfe und Unterstützung in jedem Augenblick alles geheilt werden wird.

Übernehmen Sie wieder die Verantwortung und folglich auch Ihre Macht und werden Sie zu dem Meister, der Sie bereits sind. Wenn jeder Mann, jede Frau und jedes Kind wieder die Verantwortung übernimmt, wird sich die Welt wahrhaftig in jenes Paradies verwandeln, als das sie vorgesehen war. Dies ist möglich, meine Lieben, aber nur, wenn jeder von Euch seine Rolle spielt und seine Macht wieder in Anspruch nimmt. Geht als ersten Schritt in Richtung Eurer wahrhaftigen Meisterschaft diese Verpflichtung ein. Nehmt die Meisterschaft jetzt in Anspruch!

Geben Sie alles, was Sie lernen, an Ihre Freunde, Bekannten und Eltern weiter. Lassen Sie zu, dass diese einfachen Wahrheiten sich wie ein Lauffeuer verbreiten werden. Sehen Sie, wie dieses wundervolle Licht blitzartig weitergegeben wird. Bald wird die Erde von dem wunderbaren Christuslicht, das in jedem von Euch enthalten ist, überflutet werden. Kommt, meine geliebten Regenbogen-Krieger, hebt Eure Fackeln hoch und marschiert siegessicher voran. Fürchtet Euch nicht! Denn ich bin immer bei Euch!

Je mehr Sie sich auf diesen Schlüssel konzentrieren, desto besser werden Sie verstehen, dass es wahrhaftig keine Traurigkeit, keine Verzweiflung und kein Leid auf diesem Planeten gäbe, wenn jeder wirklich die Verantwortung für jeden Gedanken, jedes Wort und jede Tat übernehmen würde.

Kapitel zwei

Schlüssel Nummer zwei: Loslassen von alten Mustern

Bevor Sie diesen Ort, an dem vollkommener Friede, Liebe und Freude herrschen, erreichen können, ist es notwendig, alte Muster loszulassen, die Ihnen nicht mehr dienlich sind. Es ist im Handumdrehen möglich, diese Muster loszulassen, die Sie seit einer Ewigkeit in Gefangenschaft gehalten haben!

Sind Sie bereit, dies zu tun? Oder möchten Sie noch ein wenig länger leiden und das Opfer dieser alten Muster sein? Wenn die Antwort auf die erste Frage ein „Ja!" ist, dann sollten Sie diese Übung machen. Sie werden erstaunt sein, wie einfach und schmerzlos dies ist. Wichtig ist, sich daran zu erinnern, dass Sie, nachdem Sie dieses alte Muster losgelassen haben, unbedingt daran GLAUBEN sollen, dass es nicht mehr vorhanden ist. Ansonsten, wenn Sie sich wieder auf das Problem konzentrieren, werden Sie das Problem wieder entstehen lassen, und die ganze Prozedur muss nochmals und abermals wiederholt werden!

Das Loslassen von alten Mustern ist eine leichte Angelegenheit. Es ist so einfach, dass Sie vielleicht an der Berechtigung dieser Übung zweifeln werden! Die Verfasserin dieses Buches kann mit jeder Zelle ihres eigenen Körpers dafür bürgen, dass es funktioniert! Sie setzt dieses Werkzeug ständig und mit großem Erfolg ein. Der Erfolg entzieht sich ihr, wenn sie die ungewollte Energie ständig durch Sorgen oder Zweifel zurückverlangt. Langsam, aber sicher beherrscht sie dies wunderbar, und sie ist bereit, diese Gaben an andere weiterzugeben, sodass auch diese an der Großartigkeit dieser Gaben teilhaben können.

Wenn Sie mitten in einem alten Muster stecken, das Sie überhaupt nicht leiden können und von dem Sie wirklich schon die Nase voll haben, sollten Sie folgendermaßen vorgehen:

1. Anerkennen Sie das Muster.

2. Sehen Sie sich den Kern des Musters an, danken Sie ihm für alles, was es Ihnen beigebracht hat, und seien Sie dankbar für alle erteilten Lektionen.

3. Nehmen Sie es als Teil Ihrer Ganzheit an und treffen Sie dann die Entscheidung, es loszulassen, und sagen Sie in Gedanken oder laut:

„Ich beschließe, dieses alte Muster von .... an meine mächtige ICH-BIN-Gegenwart zu übergeben, und glaube, dass es jetzt und für alle Ewigkeit verschwunden ist. Amen. So sei es, so geschehe es." (Dreimal wiederholen.) Rufen Sie dann die mächtige violette Flamme an, dass sie kommen und Sie mit diesem Licht umgeben und dabei sämtliche Restenergien, die Ihnen nicht mehr dienlich sind, transformieren und verwandeln möge.

Dies wird zur Folge haben, dass alle alten Muster an die Oberfläche kommen werden, damit sie nacheinander bereinigt werden können, je nachdem, wie rasch Sie diese auflösen und loswerden möchten. Manchmal kann dies ziemlich intensiv werden. Sie können auch die Meister des Lichts bitten, eine Pause einzulegen, die sie Ihnen gerne gewähren werden. Wenn Sie bereit sind, fortzufahren, bitten Sie die Meister wieder!

Die geliebten Meister, Geistführer, Lehrer und Engel sind immer an unserer Seite und warten darauf, uns unterstützen zu können. Wenn Sie Hilfe benötigen, sollten Sie sich nicht scheuen, darum zu bitten, denn sie können nur dann eingreifen, wenn Sie ihnen die Erlaubnis dazu geben. Wenn Sie um Hilfe beten, sollten

Sie immer darum bitten, dass Ihnen das Höchste und Beste und an diesem Tag zuteil werden möge. Dies ermöglicht es dem höheren Selbst, zu entscheiden, was unter diesen Umständen am besten für Sie ist.

Ein wirkliches Loslassen von alten Mustern erfolgt nur über die Vergebung von allem, sowohl in Ihrer Aura als auch in Ihrem Leben. Wenn Sie sämtlichen Leuten alles vergeben haben, werden alle Verträge aufgelöst, und dies ist „das Gesetz". (Sue hat festgestellt, dass die schwierigste Aufgabe darin besteht, sich selbst zu vergeben und sie arbeitet ständig daran.)

Vor allem sollten Sie stets daran denken, Dankbarkeit gegenüber Ihrer mächtigen ICH-BIN-Gegenwart, den Engeln, Meistern, Geistführern und Lehrern, die an Ihrer Seite verweilen und Ihnen jeden Tag helfen, diesen Weg in Richtung Erleuchtung zu beschreiten, zum Ausdruck zu bringen. Denken Sie daran, sich bei ihnen für all diese wunderbaren Geschenke, die Sie erhalten, zu bedanken. (Eine schöne Übung wäre, sich jeden Tag für alle Segnungen in Ihrem Leben, einschließlich sämtlicher Prüfungen und Strapazen, zu bedanken. Denn dies ermöglicht es Ihnen, zu wachsen und zu verstehen, was es wirklich bedeutet, ein Meister zu sein.)

Es ist so einfach, meine Lieben. Verwendet diese Instrumente so oft wie möglich, und Ihr werdet allmählich verstehen, wie wunderbar das Leben sein kann! Die

Schlüssel zum Königreich des Himmels sind einfach und zugänglich für jeden, der bereit ist, in sich zu gehen.

Wir nehmen die Schwierigkeiten wahr, die Ihr als Menschen, die schon seit Äonen auf der Erde wandeln, habt. Jetzt ist es an der Zeit, in Eure eigene Macht und Meisterschaft zu kommen und die wirkliche Bedeutung dessen, was es heißt, den Himmel auf die Erde zu bringen, zu verstehen. Jede Seele hat ihr eigenes Schicksal und einen Weg, dem es zu folgen gilt. Alles ist jederzeit in göttlicher Ordnung. Versucht niemals, Euch selbst oder andere zu etwas zu drängen. Wenn man dies tut, können wichtige Lektionen übersehen werden, die dann zu einem späteren Zeitpunkt wiederholt werden müssen. Gestattet es Spirit, Euch zu inspirieren, und hört auf Euer Herz, meine Geliebten. Dies ist der Weg nach Hause.

Wenn Ihr in diesem Himmel auf Erden wohnt, werden all die Menschen rund um Euch automatisch in diesen Zustand von Frieden, Freude, Zufriedenheit, Harmonie, Fülle und Einfachheit versetzt. Eure Schwingung ist so hoch, dass Ihr keine Worte braucht – Eure Gegenwart versetzt die Leute in Eurer unmittelbaren Umgebung in einen glückseligen Seinszustand. Seht täglich zu, wie sich dies entwickelt, und anerkennt den Christus in Euch, Eure mächtige ICH-BIN-Gegenwart, so oft wie möglich. Bringt allem, was existiert, große Dankbarkeit und tiefe Bewunderung entgegen.

Sobald Ihr den Christus in Euch anerkennen könnt, werdet Ihr in allen Dingen und Menschen, die Euch begegnen, den Christus sehen. Gestattet es Euch selbst, zu strahlen wie das helle Licht, das Ihr seid. Wenn Ihr das tut, erteilt Ihr anderen die Erlaubnis, es Euch gleichzutun. Stellt Euch vor, wie hell und wunderschön Ihr seid. Akzeptiert und anerkennt dies zu jeder Zeit.

Kapitel drei

Schlüssel Nummer drei: Vergebung

Vergebung ist wahrhaftig der Schlüssel zum Glücklichsein. Wenn ein Mensch anderen nicht vergeben kann, ist dies ein Zeichen, dass der Mensch sich selbst nicht vergeben kann. Um dies etwas verständlicher zu machen, möchten wir Ihnen das folgende Ritual schildern, das vor allem in der Gruppe sehr wirksam ist. Es kann natürlich auch von einer einzelnen Person angewandt werden.

1. Schreiben Sie zuerst alle Menschen auf, denen Sie in Ihrem Leben bis jetzt noch nicht vergeben konnten.

2. Schreiben Sie neben dem Namen auf, was Ihnen dieser Mensch angeblich angetan hat.

3. Denken Sie über diese Menschen nach und stellen Sie fest, ob Sie die Verantwortung für deren Handlungen übernehmen können. Denn in Wahrheit, meine geliebten Kinder des Lichts, kann Euch niemand etwas antun! Sie sind niemals ein Opfer. Sie erschaffen stets alles selbst, immer. Dies ist sehr ermächtigend.

4. Wenn Sie diese Verantwortung wirklich übernehmen können, dann sind Sie selbst der erste Mensch, dem Sie vergeben sollten. Dies ist normalerweise das Schwierigste. Lernen Sie, Mitgefühl für sich selbst sowie für die Fehler und die Schmerzen, die Sie sich selbst auferlegt haben, zu zeigen.

   Wenn Sie einmal sich selbst vergeben können, ist es einfach, anderen zu vergeben, denn somit wissen Sie, dass es nichts zu vergeben gibt!

   Unsere Seele erschafft für uns ständig eine Situation, in der wir lernen und wachsen können. Wenn Sie diese Wahrheit akzeptieren, wird das Leben viel einfacher werden. Es mag eine gewisse Zeit dauern, bis Sie voll und ganz die Verantwortung für alles, was Ihnen widerfährt, übernehmen können. Wenn Sie allerdings diese einfache universelle Wahrheit verstehen, liegt der Weg zur Freiheit vor Ihnen, und das Einzige, was Sie zu tun haben, ist, diesen Weg zu beschreiten!

Sämtliche Methoden und Schlüssel, die in diesem kleinen Buch erklärt werden, können von Ihnen leicht und mühelos umgesetzt werden, wenn Sie bereit sind, Ihr Herz zu öffnen, um diese äußerst wirksamen Wahrheiten zu empfangen.

5. Nachdem Sie die Verantwortung für die Handlungen und Umstände übernommen haben, die Ihnen Schmerzen bereitet haben, rufen Sie das Gesetz der Vergebung und Ihre mächtige ICH-BIN-Gegenwart an, um Ihnen alles zu vergeben, wofür Sie anderen die Schuld gegeben haben, obwohl die Schuld in Wirklichkeit bei Ihnen gelegen ist. Sagen Sie: „Ich bin das Gesetz der Vergebung und die mächtige violette Flamme der Verwandlung, die all meine Fehler, Ursache und Wirkung, Aufzeichnungen und Erinnerungen von Anbeginn der Zeit bis jetzt löscht." Seien Sie sich bewusst, dass Ihre mächtige ICH-BIN-Gegenwart in Ihnen verweilt – und dass Sie dieselbe sind. Übergeben Sie es an Ihre ICH-BIN-Gegenwart und gestatten Sie es ihr, die Kontrolle über Ihren Geist, Ihren Körper und Ihre Welt zu übernehmen und die Herrschaft über Sie zu haben. Auf diese Weise wird Ihr Leben von Augenblicken erfüllt sein, an denen Sie eine Gänsehaut bekommen. Jedes Mal, wenn Ihr Ego zum Beispiel urteilen oder eingreifen möchte, können Sie dies an Ihre ICH-BIN-Gegenwart übergeben und die ICH-BIN-Gegenwart des anderen Menschen,

über den Sie urteilen, bitten, das Kommando über die Situation zu übernehmen und hier Vollkommenheit zu erschaffen. Der Schlüssel zur Erlangung von Himmel auf Erden liegt in der Hingabe jedes einzelnen Augenblicks an Ihr höheres Selbst. Bittet und es soll Euch gegeben werden – Gott ist liebend und vergebend, und er gibt uns stets eine neue Chance. Ganz gleich, welches Gefühl Sie haben, seien Sie sich bewusst, dass Ihnen vergeben wird. Sich selbst zu vergeben, ist der Schlüssel.

6. Gehen Sie dann zu Ihrem höheren Selbst. Bitten Sie Ihre Seele um Vergebung für all den Schmerz und das Leid, das Sie sich selbst verursacht haben, und bedanken Sie sich herzlich für sämtliche Lektionen, die Sie aufgrund dieser Erfahrungen gelernt haben.

7. Wenden Sie sich dann an Ihr inneres Kind und bitten Sie es um Vergebung. Gewöhnlich beinhaltet dies eine Menge an Schmerzen und Leid. Nehmen Sie Ihr Kind in die Arme, lieben und trösten Sie es und bringen Sie ihm Mitgefühl entgegen, denn gewöhnlich liegt hier der Ursprung des Problems. Sehr oft vergessen Sie, auf die Schreie des Kindes in Ihrem Inneren zu hören.

8. Nehmen Sie sich jeden Tag Zeit, mit Ihrem inneren Kind zu sprechen, und Sie werden sein tägliches Wachstum und seine Aufregung darüber, endlich

anerkannt zu werden, erleben. Fragen Sie, was es heute gerne tun würde, und warten Sie, welche Antwort kommt!

9. Lassen Sie zu, dass Sie von Frieden und Liebe erfüllt werden. Spüren Sie die Freude, die Sie erleben, wenn Sie sich selbst vergeben, und die Freiheit, die dies mit sich bringt. Denn wenn Sie jeden Teil der menschlichen Erfahrung in Freude und vollkommener Akzeptanz für alles wirklich annehmen können, werden Sie ein Meister sein.

10. Gehen Sie dann die Liste von Leuten durch, denen Sie nicht vergeben können, und bitten Sie jeden von ihnen um Vergebung. Dies kann getan werden, indem Sie das höhere Selbst dieser Person anrufen. Oder, wenn Sie es für notwendig halten, sagen Sie es ihnen persönlich. Besser wäre noch, jedem von ihnen einen Brief zu schreiben, in dem Sie bestätigen, wie Sie sich gefühlt haben, und all Ihre Gefühle zum Ausdruck bringen.
    Diese Leute haben nur ihre Rolle im Spiel gespielt, damit jeder von Ihnen seine Lektion lernen konnte. Vergeben und danken Sie diesen Personen dafür, dass sie diese Rolle gespielt haben. Und zum Schluss sollten Sie sie um Vergebung bitten.

Dieser Brief sollte in einem Ritual verbrannt werden. Dies ist eine sehr machtvolle Übung. Es gibt unzählige Möglichkeiten dafür, die „Wahrheit" in jeder Situation herauszufinden. Wenn Sie sich selbst gegenüber wirklich ehrlich sind, sollten Sie auch nach jeder Beschuldigung dazu fähig sein, „Ich auch!" zu sagen.

Wenn sich etwas ereignet hat, sind Sie oft so gekränkt und bestürzt über das Ereignis, dass Sie Schwierigkeiten damit haben, es loszulassen und zu vergeben. Lassen Sie bitte nicht zu, dass Sie selbst noch länger leiden. Verwenden Sie diese Instrumente und befreien Sie sich selbst von den Fesseln der Vergangenheit. Es ist nun an der Zeit für Sie, in Freude und Glückseligkeit sowie im Augenblick zu leben. Keine Schmerzen und kein Leid mehr. Nach diesem Ritual ist es ratsam, buchstäblich alles wegzuspülen, entweder unter einem Wasserfall, im Ozean oder in der Dusche.

Rufen Sie jede Nacht vor dem Schlafengehen das Gesetz der Vergebung an, um jegliche negative Gedanken, Worte oder Taten, die Sie begangen haben, zu löschen und zu transformieren. Dies wird weitere karmische Schuld für die Zukunft eliminieren. Diese Bitte sollte selbstverständlich, immer mit größtmöglicher Aufrichtigkeit und wirklicher Reue geäußert werden.

Dies sind äußerst einfache universelle Wahrheiten, an die sich die Menschheit erinnern sollte. Sie sollten den Kindern des goldenen Zeitalters beigebracht werden, während sie noch klein genug sind, um während dem Aufwachsen diese Wahrheiten zu erlernen, zu kennen und zu akzeptieren. Wenn ihnen diese Fakten beigebracht werden, werden sie nicht mehr all den Schmerz und das Leid durchmachen müssen. Es obliegt nun Ihnen, diese Weisheit weiterzugeben.

Kapitel vier

Universelle Wahrheiten

Wenn den Kindern ihre wahre Identität verwehrt wird, verlieren sie ihr Gespür dafür, wer sie in Wirklichkeit sind. Hierin besteht die Gefahr. Es ist absolut notwendig, dass alle Menschen ihre Göttlichkeit verstehen und sich damit identifizieren können.

Es wird im Unterbewusstsein immer einige unbekannte Talente geben. Wenn man den Kindern die Freiheit lässt, sich selbst auszudrücken, wie sie möchten, wird es ihnen ermöglicht, sich wie eine wunderschöne Rose in der Mittagssonne zu entfalten, ohne Angst davor, gerügt zu werden. Ermutigen Sie die Kinder dazu, ihren Träumen zu folgen, ganz gleich, wie verrückt sie auch erscheinen mögen. Die Kinder wissen, was das Richtige für sie ist und was ihre Seele zu lernen hat. Wenn man ihnen den Raum und die Freiheit zugesteht, sich zu entfalten, wie sie es in ihrer eigenen Zeit möchten, werden Sie wahrhaftig erstaunt sein! Ehren Sie die großen Wesen, die die Kinder sind.

Es gibt viele, die diese Wahrheit verleugnen, doch bald wird alles offenbart werden, und sämtliche Dinge, die nicht in Übereinstimmung mit dem Göttlichen sind, werden keinen Platz mehr haben. Alles wird offenbart werden, und die Wahrheit wird allen bekannt sein, ob es den anderen gefallen wird oder nicht. Universelle Wahrheiten können nicht verleugnet oder verändert werden, sie sind ganz einfach vorhanden.

Wenn in Ihrer Familie oder Ihren Beziehungen zu Freunden oder Kollegen Schwierigkeiten auftauchen, sollten Sie sich immer ansehen, was Ihnen dieser Mensch widerspiegelt. Sie sollten jederzeit sich selbst und anderen gegenüber sehr ehrlich sein. Darin ist das wunderbare Geschenk des Wachstums enthalten. Wenn man die Schwierigkeiten unbeachtet lässt, werden sie bestehen bleiben, bis Sie bereit sind, sie wirklich in Augenschein zu nehmen.

Meine lieben und geliebten Kinder, wir wissen, dass es nicht immer leicht ist, diese alten Muster loszulassen, die die Menschheit seit tausenden Jahren ausgespielt hat. Doch Ihr habt nun die wunderbare Gelegenheit, sie mit Leichtigkeit und Anmut loszulassen. Seht jedes Muster als eine Lernerfahrung und nehmt es als einen Freund an, dem Ihr über den Kopf gewachsen seid.

Liebt und akzeptiert sie und lasst sie nacheinander los. Ihr werdet erstaunt sein, wie viel Licht Ihr spüren werdet! Nehmt Euch selbst an und liebt Euch selbst. Dies sind die Schlüssel, die Euch auf Eurem Weg nachhause helfen sollen.

Wir wissen, dass das Ego seine Opferrolle manchmal nicht aufgeben möchte, doch wir empfehlen Euch dringend, es auf einen Versuch ankommen zu lassen und Euch anzusehen, wie einfach dies ist. Das Ego hat stets Angst vor etwas Neuem und Unbekanntem. Dies ist auch der Grund, warum es ständig Widerstand leistet.

Die universellen Wahrheiten

Selbstbeherrschung bedeutet nichts anderes, als die universellen Wahrheiten jederzeit zu verstehen und anzuwenden. Nachdem so viele Jahre ohne dieses Wissen verstrichen sind, ist es wesentlich, diese Grundregeln zu lernen und zu akzeptieren:

1. Was man aussendet, kehrt zurück.

2. Lieben Sie Ihren Nächsten wie sich selbst.

3. Reagieren Sie nicht auf die Handlungen Ihres Nächsten, halten Sie auch die andere Wange hin.

4. Sie bekommen das, was Sie denken.

5. Sie sind in jedem Augenblick ein Schöpfer und suchen sich Ihr Leben aus, wie Sie es haben möchten.

6. Sie sind niemals ein Opfer – Sie erschaffen jede Situation, um etwas daraus zu lernen.

7. Verantwortung – übernehmen Sie Verantwortung für jeden Gedanken, jedes Wort und jede Tat.

8. Vergebung – vergeben Sie sich selbst und anderen.

9. Urteilen – urteilen Sie nicht über sich selbst oder andere.

10. Verurteilen – verurteilen Sie sich selbst und andere nicht.

11. Glauben Sie an sich selbst und andere.

12. Dankbarkeit in jeder Situation.

13. Die Dinge, denen wir uns widersetzen, bleiben bestehen.

14. Nehmen Sie jede Situation in Ihrem Leben, wie sie im Augenblick ist, als vollkommen hin.

Inmitten des Chaos, welches in der Welt gegenwärtig herrscht, ist es möglich, im Inneren Frieden zu finden. Darin ist ein sehr wesentlicher Schlüssel enthalten. Wenn Sie in jeder Situation Frieden bewahren können, sind Sie wahrhaftig ein Meister. Wenn Sie dazu fähig sind, in Frieden und angstfrei zu bleiben, sind Sie ein Meister. Habe Geduld, mit Dir selbst, meine Liebe. Rom ist auch nicht an einem Tag erbaut worden. Habe Mitgefühl und Verständnis und liebe Dich selbst und andere. Dies ist so wesentlich.

Als Christus vor zweitausend Jahren auf der Erde wandelte, machten ihm all diese Versuchungen zu schaffen, die er zu meistern hatte. Jedes Mal, wenn Ihr in die Materie zurückkehrt, kommt ein Schleier herunter, und Ihr vergesst buchstäblich alles, was Euch in anderen Reichen bekannt war. Der Lernprozess beginnt wieder einmal, mit dem Hauptaugenmerk auf bestimmte Lektionen, die Ihr in diesem Leben bewältigen sollt. Vollkommenheit auf Erden ist mehr oder weniger unmöglich. Selbst den Heiligen fiel dies schwer! Denkt daran, dass Ihr zu jeder Zeit Eurem Herzen folgen sollt, und dann wird die Wahrheit offenbart werden.

Meditation und Visualisierung
Quelle der Jugend und Verjüngung

Atmen Sie in das Zentrum Ihres Herzens ein und spüren Sie die Quelle der Liebe in Ihrem Inneren. Bitten Sie darum, dass in Ihrem Herzen die Quelle der Gesundheit, Jugend und Verjüngung hervorsprudeln möge. Spüren Sie, wie diese Quelle kristalliner Energie in Ihnen hochsteigt und wie ein Champagner in jeder Zelle Ihres Körpers prickelt. Spüren Sie, wie jede Zelle aufspringt und in kristallines Licht verwandelt wird.

Wenn Sie das Gefühl haben, dass dieser Prozess vollständig ist, bitten Sie die mächtige violette Flamme, zu erscheinen und jegliche Restenergien, die Ihnen nicht mehr von Nutzen sind, umzuwandeln. Spüren und sehen Sie, wie Sie in dieser wunderschönen violetten Flamme eingehüllt sind, und bedanken Sie sich herzlich für diese wundervollen Geschenke. Es ist eine Tatsache, dass der Jungbrunnen in jedem von uns enthalten ist. Bei ständiger Anwendung und durch den Beschluss: ICH BIN der vollkommene jugendliche und gesunde Körper, werden Sie sich verjüngen.

Es ist so wichtig, die Essenz Ihres Wesens anzuerkennen. Bald werden Sie die Ergebnisse bemerken, und Ihre Freunde werden sich zu Ihrer Jugendlichkeit äußern! Versucht es, meine Lieben, es wird mit Sicherheit funktionieren. In den kommenden Jahren wird es kein Älterwerden und keinen Tod, wie Ihr ihn kennt, geben. Alles wird bewusst und in göttlicher Übereinstimmung mit dem Schicksal Eurer Seele geschehen. Dies mag für einige von Euch schwer zu verstehen sein, aber ich versichere Euch, meine Geliebten, dass dies die Wahrheit ist.

Um die Wahrheit zu identifizieren, braucht Ihr nur in Euer Herz zu gehen und spüren, ob es richtig ist oder nicht. Ihr werdet es augenblicklich wissen. Lasst Euch nicht von Eurem Verstand davon überzeugen, dass es vernünftiger wäre, dieses oder jenes zu tun! Das erste Gefühl ist intuitiv und kommt von Spirit. Hört auf diese Worte des Wissens, denn sie enthalten immer die Wahrheit.

Kapitel fünf

Lernen Sie, mit Ihren Emotionen umzugehen

Wenn Sie sich als Opfer einer bestimmten Situation fühlen, so liegt das daran, dass Sie ab dem Zeitpunkt, an dem Sie die Energie ausgesandt haben, in einem Zeitraffer waren und die wiederkehrende Energie scheint Sie dann aus heiterem Himmel zu treffen. Sie behaupten: „Es ist unmöglich, dass ich mit dieser Situation etwas zu tun habe!“ Natürlich haben Sie damit etwas zu tun, sonst wäre sie nicht erschaffen worden!

Bei der Lektion geht es darum, jedes Wort und jeden Gedanken Ihrerseits zu beobachten. Überprüfen Sie sich selbst, und wenn Sie einen Gedanken haben, der eine nicht gerade hohe Schwingung hat, löschen Sie ihn, indem Sie einfach nur „löschen, löschen“ sagen, und beginnen Sie von vorne. Wenn Sie in jedem

Augenblick bewusst handeln, wird sich Ihr Leben einfacher gestalten.

Denken Sie daran, für sich selbst in jedem Augenblick Liebe und Mitgefühl aufzubringen, auch wenn Sie die Tiefe der Verzweiflung erreicht haben. Wenn Sie sich wütend oder traurig, deprimiert oder krank fühlen, sollten Sie sich selbst annehmen. Akzeptieren Sie, wie Sie sich fühlen, und nehmen Sie die Erfahrung an. Laufen Sie nicht vor dem Gefühl davon und ignorieren Sie es auch nicht, ansonsten wird es stets wiederkehren, bis Sie es bewältigt haben. Akzeptieren Sie, dass an all diesen, Emotionen nichts „falsch" ist. Sie alle sind ein Teil des Ganzen. Lieben Sie diese Emotionen als Teil der Polaritätserfahrung. Die Dinge, denen wir uns widersetzen, bleiben bestehen!

Gott gab Ihnen all diese Gefühle und Emotionen, damit Sie vielleicht etwas daraus lernen würden – verwenden Sie diese als Instrumente, um herauszufinden, ob etwas nicht übereinstimmt. Was sollen Sie aus dieser Reaktion lernen? Wenn Sie eine Reaktion auf etwas haben, sollen Sie wissen, dass dies Ihre Reaktion ist und dass Sie daraus etwas lernen sollen!

Allmählich werden Sie lernen, mehr Selbstdisziplin aufzubringen, indem Sie nicht zulassen, dass Sie von Emotionen, die Ihnen nicht mehr dienlich sind, zermürbt werden. Es wird Ihnen gelingen, zu jeder Zeit ausgeglichener, friedvoller und glücklicher zu sein. Die Verwendung der verzehrenden violetten Flamme und des goldenen Lichtstrahls wird Ihnen dabei helfen, Ihre Emotionalkörper von sämtlichen schädlichen Energien zu reinigen, und zwar vom Anbeginn der Zeit bis jetzt.

Wenn Sie sich das nächste Mal deprimiert fühlen, fragen Sie sich selbst, warum? Wodurch wird dies verursacht? Gehen Sie dem Problem auf den Grund und gestatten Sie sich selbst, wirklich zu spüren, was Sie hier durchmachen. Das wird Ihnen helfen, dies loszulassen, wie wir in den vorherigen Kapiteln beschrieben haben. Sie brauchen keine Schuldgefühle zu haben, weil Sie verärgert oder wütend waren, bleiben Sie nur bei der Energie und spüren Sie, woher sie kommt, damit Sie diese Energie dann loslassen können.

Wir bitten Euch, bei gechannelten Botschaften stets kritisch zu sein. Dort draußen existieren so viele widersprüchliche Informationen. Die Urteilskraft ist eine der größten Lektionen, die Ihr zu lernen habt.

Wir bieten der Menschheit in dieser Zeit unsere Dienste an, um jeden Einzelnen von Euch dabei zu unterstützen, Euren Aufstieg gemeinsam mit dem Aufstieg Eurer geliebten Mutter Erde zu erlangen. Die Zeit nähert sich buchstäblich ihrem Ende, und es wird das neue goldene Zeitalter in seiner ganzen Pracht anbrechen, damit es von allen gesehen werden kann.

Viele Tage voller Schönheit und Lobpreisung stehen Euch bevor. Werdet Ihr diese wundersame Zukunft als Eure Zukunft hinnehmen? Durch das gottgegebene Geschenk des freien Willens liegt es heute und in Zukunft stets an Euch, zu entscheiden, an welcher Art von Zukunft Ihr teilhaben möchtet. Wenn Ihr Euch für Vollkommenheit, Schönheit, Frieden, Glück und Liebe entscheidet, dann werdet Ihr genau das bekommen! Wenn Ihr Euch Eure Zukunft schwierig und voller Probleme, Hunger, Erdbeben, Katastrophen vorstellt, werdet Ihr genau das erschaffen.

Dies liegt gänzlich an Euren Herzenswünschen, denn die Zeit läuft ab und das neue Zeitalter wird Euch blitzartig bevorstehen. Alles wird im Handumdrehen offenbart werden und bis zu dieser Zeit werdet Ihr verstanden haben, dass es an Euch liegt, das zu erschaffen, was Ihr jetzt möchtet, sodass die Vollkommenheit Eurer Welt im Handumdrehen vorhanden sein wird, wenn die Zeit gekommen ist.

Seid im Frieden, meine Lieben, und wisset, dass ICH immer bei Euch bin und im Zentrum Eurer Herzen bleibe und darauf warte, von Euch angerufen zu werden, um Euch auf jede mir mögliche Weise zu helfen. Die aufgestiegenen Meister bieten Euch allesamt ihre treue Unterstützung an, wenn Ihr darum bittet.

Es ist notwendig, um etwas zu bitten, denn wir greifen niemals unbefugt in die Wünsche anderer ein. Wir danken jedem Einzelnen von Euch für Eure aufrichtige Arbeit und Eure ergebenen Dienste an das Licht und dafür, dass Ihr Euch selbst und die Menschheit von den Fesseln der gesamten menschlichen Schöpfung befreit. Wir bringen der mächtigen ICH-BIN-Gegenwart in jedem von Euch Bewunderung entgegen und bestärken Euch, mit der Reinigung Eures Körpers, Eures Geistes und Eurer Welten durch die verzehrende violette Flamme fortzufahren.

Ruft das Gesetz der Vergebung aufrichtig an, und es wird Euch alles in diesem Leben und aus sämtlichen Leben, von Anbeginn Eurer Inkarnationen bis jetzt, vergeben werden. Erlaubt es Euch selbst, in diesen mächtigen magischen Lichtkreis eingehüllt zu werden, der sämtliche unharmonische Energie fernhält und Euch davor schützt, was die göttliche Vollkommenheit, Liebe und Harmonie eintreten lässt. Seht, wie Ihr jeden Tag von der mächtigen violetten Flamme erfüllt und von einem Lichtstrahl umgeben werdet, und ruft zuerst stets das Gesetz der Vergebung an. Auf diese Weise, meine Lieben, seid Ihr für immer von Euren Fehlern befreit. Ihr braucht die Auswirkungen des Karmas nicht mehr länger zu erleiden. Alles wird durch den fortwährenden Einsatz der folgenden Instrumente erleichtert.

Schritte, um Körper, Geist, Aura und die Welt von unharmonischen Energien zu reinigen:

1. Rufen Sie das Gesetz der Vergebung an und bringen Sie Ihrer mächtigen ICH-BIN-Gegenwart Dank und Bewunderung entgegen. Lenken Sie die Energie Ihres mächtigen Meisterselbst (Ihrer ICH-BIN-Gegenwart), um sämtliche Fehler, die Sie begangen haben, zu beheben und zu ändern. Auf diese Weise können Sie sich von der Reaktion der lieblosen Gedanken, Worte und Taten befreien, die Sie bewusst und unbewusst geäußert bzw. begangen haben.

   Verwenden Sie dieses Geschenk und Werkzeug fortwährend im Laufe jedes Tages. Jedes Mal, wenn Sie einen lieblosen Gedanken betreffend jemand anderen hegen, reinigen Sie ihn. Und bitten Sie um Vergebung, sobald Sie sich dessen bewusst werden.

   Am Ende des Tages sollten Sie dasselbe nochmals tun und darum bitten, dass Ihnen alle Fehler vergeben werden mögen, selbst jene, derer Sie sich noch nicht gewahr sind. Wir versprechen Euch, dass Ihr, wenn Ihr diese wundervollen Geschenke verwendet, im wahrsten Sinne des Wortes allmählich ein Leben voller Freude und Freiheit erfahren werdet.

2. Rufen Sie die mächtige violette Flamme an, um sämtliche schädlichen Energien in Ihrem Geist, Ihrem Körper und Ihrer Welt zu verzehren. Stellen Sie sich vor, wie Sie diese wunderbare violette Flamme mit ihrer Gegenwart einhüllt, von Ihren Füßen bis zu Ihrer Kopfspitze und weiter hinaus. Und wie sie dabei jegliche unharmonische Energie transformiert und umwandelt.

   Das bedeutet, dass alle negativen Gedankenformen und Urteile, die Sie in das Universum seit Anbeginn der Zeit ausgesandt haben, allmählich, Tag für Tag (je nachdem, mit welcher Ernsthaftigkeit Sie dieses wunderbare Werkzeug einsetzen) in reines Licht umgewandelt werden. Ihre ganze Aura, Ihr Körper und Ihr Geist werden gereinigt. Schließlich werden Sie eines Morgens aufwachen und ein sauberes Haus haben, in dem Ihre mächtige ICH-BIN-Gegenwart wohnen kann. Dann kann SIE Ihr Leben immer näher betreten. Sobald SIE sieht, dass Sie die mächtige Energie, die verfügbar wird, nicht missbrauchen, werden Sie dazu fähig sein, viele wundervolle Geschenke von Spirit zu nutzen, doch zuerst müssen Sie in Haus und Hof Ihren Frühjahrsputz machen.

3. Rufen Sie die mächtige ICH-BIN-Gegenwart an, um Sie mittels dem goldenen Lichtstrahl zu behüten und zu beschützen.

4. Sagen Sie der mächtigen ICH-BIN-Gegenwart, was Sie möchten: „Ich BIN gesund, wohlhabend, glücklich etc." Verfügen Sie dies ernsthaft, jeden Tag, immer, wenn Sie daran denken. Jedes Mal, wenn Sie ICH BIN sagen, rufen Sie die GOTTES-Gegenwart in Ihrem Herzen und Ihrem Wesen an. Sie bestätigen damit der Gegenwart, was Sie möchten. Seien Sie vorsichtig mit dem, was Sie sagen – wenn Sie sagen, „Ich bin krank", raten Sie mal, was die ICH-BIN-Gegenwart denkt, was Sie möchten – ein wenig mehr von der Krankheit!
   Sagen Sie stattdessen: „Ich bin in jeder Zelle meines Körpers gesund. Die Illusion der Krankheit hat keine Macht über mich." Ganz gleich, was es auch sein mag, schenken Sie dem keine Aufmerksamkeit und rufen Sie die ICH-BIN-Gegenwart an, um über Ihnen zu wachen, damit keine unharmonische Energie eindringen kann!
   Die Energie von Gott, die ICH BIN Gegenwart, ist neutral. Durch unsere Gedanken geben wir ihr eine positive oder negative Note.

5. Erinnern Sie sich daran, dass Sie der Schöpfer Ihrer Welt sind. Beobachten Sie, was Sie denken, sagen und tun! Wenn Sie sich auf große Fülle konzentrieren, werden Sie das erhalten (sofern Ihre unbewussten Gedanken diese Anordnung nicht rückgängig machen). Das ist das göttliche Gesetz.

6. Rufen Sie Ihre höheren Mentalkörper an, um über Ihrer Welt zu wachen und nichts anderes als die Wahrheit zuzulassen. Geben Sie von Menschen erschaffener Disharmonie etc. keine Macht.

7. Rufen Sie die aufgestiegenen Meister an, um Ihnen zu helfen, wenn Sie Schwierigkeiten damit haben, sich selbst und Ihre Emotionen zu beherrschen. Bitten Sie diese, Ihnen ihre mächtige magische Substanz zu senden, um Ihren Geist, Ihren Körper und Ihre Welt mit dieser Substanz zu erfüllen, was es Ihnen ermöglicht, tagtäglich den aufgestiegenen Meistern ähnlicher zu werden. Dies sind wahrhaftige Segnungen des Göttlichen, meine Liebe / mein Lieber. Verwenden Sie diese Instrumente in Ihrem Leben, um Ihr Leben zu verbessern und Ihre ewige Freiheit zu erlangen – den jetzigen Aufstieg Ihrer menschlichen Gestalt!

Leben Sie in Dankbarkeit für all diese mächtigen Geschenke der Anmut.

Was mit der Energie, die wir aussenden, geschieht

Eine Veranschaulichung dafür, was mit der Energie, die wir aussenden geschieht, ob positiv oder negativ:

Sie		**Andere**
Liebevoller Gedanke an	⟶	einen Freund
Liebevolle Energie von	⟵	einem Freund
Urteil, Kritik, Beschuldigung und Verurteilung an	⟶	jemanden
Urteilende Energie von	⟵	jemandem

1. Schenken Sie den Fehlern anderer Leute keine Beachtung.

2. Nehmen Sie nur die ICH-BIN-Gegenwart in jedem Menschen wahr.

3. Geben Sie unharmonischer Energie keine Macht.

4. Gott hat kein Interesse an den Fehlern des äußeren Selbst.

5. Das, worauf Sie Ihre Aufmerksamkeit richten, wird von Ihnen angezogen.

Welche Qualität dies auch haben mag, es kehrt in umso stärkerer Form wieder zurück.

Wenn Sie Ihre Gedanken auf eine Sache oder eine gewisse Qualität in einem anderen Menschen, einem Ort oder einer Sache konzentrieren, senden Sie eine Botschaft an das Universum, dass Sie zu dieser Energie hingezogen werden sollen. Das Universum reagiert immer und sendet Ihnen vieles zu, das Sie erfahren sollen – bis Sie genug davon haben und nach Vergebung schreien!

Der Schlüssel zu Ihrer Freiheit liegt genau darin: Wenn Sie die Bedeutung Ihrer urteilenden Gedanken begreifen und wie sich dies auf Sie selbst und andere auswirkt, wird das Leben um so vieles einfacher! Je aufmerksamer Sie sind und je mehr Sie über die Fehler von Ihnen und anderen nachdenken, desto mehr bekommen Sie von genau derselben Energie zurück.

Bringen Sie Mitgefühl für sich selbst und andere auf, denn Sie alle quälen sich mit den gleichen Streitfragen, Glaubenssystemen und Problemen herum. Schicken Sie jedem, der Ihnen begegnet, Liebe und Mitgefühl und Dankbarkeit für alles, was er Ihnen widerspiegelt, und lassen Sie sämtliche Beurteilungen los. Wenn Sie damit beginnen, sich auf das Gute zu konzentrieren, das Sie in allem und jedem sehen, und für alles, was Sie erfahren, dankbar sind, werden Sie allmählich diese wunderbare Energie immer mehr genießen. Probieren Sie es aus, es wird Ihnen gefallen!

Stellen Sie sich alle Menschen aus Ihrer Umgebung in einem prächtigen, weißgoldenen Lichtstrahl vor, der ausschließlich von Vollkommenheit, Freude, Frieden, Glück, Gesundheit, bedingungsloser Liebe und Fülle umgeben ist. Selbst wenn sich diese Menschen beschweren, können Sie sie bitten, einen Augenblick lang innezuhalten und sich auf das zu konzentrieren, wofür sie in ihrem Leben dankbar sein sollten.

Helfen Sie ihnen dabei, negative Gedanken in liebevolle positive Affirmationen umzuwandeln. Dies ist die netteste Sache, die Sie für einen Menschen tun können. Bemitleiden Sie die Menschen nicht wegen ihrer Probleme und helfen Sie ihnen stattdessen, ihre Wahrnehmung zu ändern, und dann werden sich die Dinge ändern.

Wenn Sie sich konzentrieren und jede Situation, jeden Menschen und jeden Ort als vollkommen akzeptieren, geben Sie ihnen die Gelegenheit, vollkommen zu werden. Die Wahrnehmung verwandelt sich dann in Vollkommenheit. Ganz gleich, wie verwirrend das Leben manchmal auch sein mag, nehmen Sie alles als vollkommen hin, und es wird vollkommen werden. Seien Sie sich bewusst, dass diese herausfordernde Erfahrung genau das ist, was Sie brauchen, um Ihre Lektionen zu lernen, auch wenn dies zeitweise etwas schmerzlich oder traurig sein mag.

Glauben und Vertrauen bedeutet zu lieben, ganz gleich, um welchen Preis, ganz gleich, ob es wie ein Versagen oder eine Täuschung seitens anderer aussieht, ganz gleich, ob es wie ein Angriff aussieht. Wie kann der Arm das Bein angreifen oder das Auge das Herz angreifen? In diesem einen Wesen ist alles Freiheit, Freude und Zufriedenheit. Wir alle sind ein Wesen und erleben uns offensichtlich als getrennt! Alles ist stets eine Widerspiegelung von Teilen unseres Selbst.

Als wir Susan neulich die Sache mit der Vollkommenheit erklärten, wurde ihr klar, dass sie sich stets so bemühte, „vollkommen" zu sein. Dabei konzentrierte sie sich ständig auf ihre Fehler und nicht auf das, was sie bereits erreicht hatte. Sie machte sich selbst das Leben schwer, indem sie sich selbst und ihre Situationen im Leben bewertete und verurteilte.

Eines Abends dämmerte ihr eine Erkenntnis und sie verstand schließlich, dass alles vollkommen sein würde, wenn sie es als vollkommen akzeptieren würde – dann wäre es vollkommen. Alles ist jederzeit vollkommen. Ein spezielles Gebet für die Vollkommenheit finden Sie am Ende dieses Buches.

Wir möchten, dass Ihr versteht, dass es von großer Bedeutung ist, jeden Gedanken, jedes Wort und jede Tat zu beobachten. Beobachtet Euch selbst in jeder Minute des Tages, und jedes Mal, wenn Ihr ein Urteil trefft, sollt Ihr das Gesetz der Vergebung anrufen und Eurem Meisterselbst befehlen, all die falschen Gedanken zu korrigieren und zu verändern.

Dies ist die einzige Art und Weise, wie wir in diesem ständigen Kreis des Lebens unsere Freiheit erlangen können. Verwenden Sie die mächtige violette Flamme und bitten Sie sie, sämtliche unharmonische Energien in Ihnen und um Sie herum, in Ihrem Zuhause, an Ihrem Arbeitsplatz etc. zu transformieren.

Im Laufe der Äonen haben Sie durch stetige Kritik, Schuld, Beurteilung von Ihnen selbst und anderen viel Geröll angehäuft. Ihre Aura ist voll von all diesen Gedanken und alten Glaubenssystemen Aus diesem Grund können wir nicht oft genug betonen, dass Ihr immerzu das Gesetz der Vergebung, die reinigende violette Flamme und den mächtigen goldenen Lichtstrahl anrufen sollt. Rufen Sie diese an, um Sie zu beschützen, und rufen Sie die mächtige ICH-BIN-Gegenwart an, um über Ihrem Geist, Ihren Gedanken, Ihrer Welt und Ihrem Zuhause zu wachen und somit jegliche disharmonische Energie aus Ihrem Leben fernzuhalten.

Sue hat eine wunderbare persönliche Geschichte zu erzählen, die sie hier gerne einbringen möchte. Es freut uns sehr, dass sie bereit ist, dies an Euch weiterzugeben, und da wir uns sicher sind, dass diese Geschichte von einem Freund stammt, wird es Euch helfen, den gesamten Prozess viel leichter zu verstehen.

Wir übersiedelten in ein wunderschönes Haus in Olinda, auf der Insel Maui. Dort hatten wir uns um neun Katzen und drei Hunde zu kümmern. Mir fiel bald auf, dass zwei Kater die ganze Zeit über die Fenster und Türen anspritzten. Die meiste Zeit über war ich relativ geduldig, doch meine Frustration nahm zu.

Ich fragte Spirit immerzu nach einer Lösung oder einer Erklärung für dieses Verhalten. Es erfolgte keine Reaktion, stattdessen wurden die Dinge noch schlimmer. Ich bat um einen Traum und erlebte zwei sehr deutliche Bilder, die mir verrieten, dass ich den seelischen Ballast anderer Leute auffing und reinigte.

Ich bemerkte fortwährend, dass ich mich jedes Mal, wenn jemand in unser Haus kam, am nächsten Tag schlecht fühlte. Eines Tages wachte ich schließlich auf und schlug aufs Geratewohl die ‚I AM Discourses' (dt. ICH-BIN-Diskurse) von Saint Germain auf, und hier fand ich schließlich auch meine Antwort. Nachdem ich die Seiten immer wieder durchgelesen hatte, erkannte ich mit jeder Zelle meines Wesens, dass jeder einzelne negative, urteilende oder kritisierende Gedanke, den ich bezüglich jemand anderen gehegt hatte, wieder zu mir zurückkam, um aufgearbeitet zu werden!

In den Träumen räumte ich ständig die Unordnung anderer Leute auf. Ich erkannte, dass ich dies schon die längste Zeit über für meine eigene Familie tat. Sobald ich in jemandem einen Charakterzug erkannt hatte, den ich nicht mochte, wurde ich mit noch mehr Aufräumarbeiten überhäuft! Ich hatte in meinem Leben schon vieles aufgeräumt und dachte, dass es nun genug sei, doch es hörte nicht auf.

Wenige Tage später verstand ich eine weitere symbolische Bedeutung der Träume. Jedes Mal, wenn mir jemand ‚seine Probleme' anvertraute, versuchte ich unbewusst, sie zu lösen. Ich suchte ständig nach einer Lösung für seine Probleme!

Obwohl ich es gut meinte und ihnen aufrichtig helfen wollte, nahm ich ihnen dadurch ihre Lektionen ab. Ich nahm ihnen ihre Lernerfahrung ab und belastete mich selbst mit noch mehr Reinigungs- und Säuberungsarbeiten.

An dem Tag, an dem ich dies begriff, war ich sehr dankbar, wieder einmal eine große Lektion erteilt zu bekommen: Wir können die Probleme anderer nicht für sie ‚beheben'. Wir können ihnen einen Rat geben, wenn wir gefragt werden, doch dann soll dieser Mensch die ganze Angelegenheit mit nach Hause nehmen, und wir sollen sie nicht mit nach Hause nehmen. Wir müssen es jedem Einzelnen gestatten, seine Lektionen zu lernen. Wir können und sollten ihnen das nicht abnehmen. Wenn wir weiterhin versuchen, dies zu tun, werden wir irgendwann vielleicht krank, weil wir uns selbst noch mehr negative Energie aufgeladen haben.

Ich weiß, dass diese alten Angewohnheiten jetzt endlich aufgelöst wurden. Ich wurde sofort noch einer Prüfung unterzogen, um zu sehen, ob ich es verstanden hatte: Harry, mein Mann, saß neben mir und ging daran, sich eine Zigarette anzuzünden! Ich ertappte mich selbst beim Gedanken: ‚Oh, ich wünschte, er würde neben mir nicht rauchen. Ich hasse diesen Gestank.'

Mein nächstes Urteil war bereits gefällt. Rasch rief ich das Gesetz der Vergebung an, um den Gedanken und die Auswirkungen, die dieser haben würde, zu reinigen. So einfach fällt man Urteile, ohne dabei überhaupt zu erkennen, dass man ein Urteil gefällt hat. Ich beobachte mich selbst nun ständig und weiß, dass dies die einzige Möglichkeit ist, wie ich selbst frei werden kann! Schenken Sie den Problemen und Handlungen anderer keine Beachtung, schenken Sie nur sich selbst Beachtung.

Ich war verzückt vor Freude und Dankbarkeit gegenüber meiner ICH-BIN-Gegenwart, den Meistern,

Lehrern, Engeln und Geistführern. Ich hatte endlich die Bedeutung aller Träume und das Verhalten der Katze verstanden.

Ich rannte herum und sang: ‚Ich bin frei, ich bin frei!' und ich konnte es nicht erwarten, die Geschichte in diesem Buch zu erzählen. Alles im Universum ist auf so wundervolle Weise ins Werk gesetzt. Alles ist jederzeit vollkommen. Das erstaunt mich ohne Ende!

Kapitel sechs

Schlüssel Nummer vier: Urteilen und Verurteilen

Über das Urteilen, Kritisieren und Verurteilen wurde bereits ausgiebig diskutiert. Hierbei handelt es sich wirklich um die Wurzel allen Übels. Wenn diese Dinge aus der menschlichen Schöpfung beseitigt werden könnten, wäre das Leben auf der Erde eine ganz andere Erfahrung.

Wir sollten verstehen, dass wir, wenn wir andere kritisieren, in Wahrheit uns selbst kritisieren. Denn wir alle sind eins und das, was wir im anderen sehen, ist stets in uns selbst gegenwärtig. Verstehen Sie dies voll und ganz?

Jedes Mal, wenn Sie bezüglich jemandem unharmonische Energie sehen oder verspüren, sollten Sie beiseite treten und sich selbst genau betrachten. Wenn Sie ehrlich sind, werden Sie in gewisser Weise die Gegenwart dieser Qualität in sich selbst bestätigen können. Es mag vielleicht in einem gegensätzlichen Zusammenhang stehen, aber in gewisser Weise spiegelt Ihnen das andere Wesen etwas wider.

Bedenken Sie, dass all dies Teil des Planes ist. Wenn Sie keine Freunde hätten, die Ihnen widerspiegeln, was Ihnen an sich selbst missfällt, wie könnten Sie diese Fehler dann korrigieren? Es ist einfach, sobald Sie einmal anerkannt haben, dass das, was Sie in jemand anderem sehen, nur eine Reflektion von einem Teil Ihres eigenen Wesens ist. Es ist auch sehr ermächtigend, wenn man sagen kann: „Ja, das stimmt, ich tue mir dies selbst bzw. anderen an."

Bedanken Sie sich herzlich für dieses Geschenk und lassen Sie dieses alte Muster los, wie in Kapitel zwei veranschaulicht. Dies ist eine sehr machtvolle Übung, und sie kann kontinuierlich angewandt werden, um alte Muster, Gewohnheiten und Glaubenssysteme loszulassen. Lassen Sie alles los, was Ihnen nicht mehr dienlich ist. Wenn es weiterhin auftaucht, sollten Sie es lieben, akzeptieren und loslassen, bis es schließlich für immer verschwunden ist! Sie müssen auf die mächtige ICH-BIN-Gegenwart vertrauen, dass diese es Ihnen abgenommen hat, ansonsten werden Sie es zurückrufen, bis Sie es dann schließlich loslassen können. „Lass los und überlasse es Gott", sagen wir Susan jeden Tag.

Manche alten Muster sind harte Angelegenheiten, die schon seit mehreren Leben andauern und sich fortsetzen werden, bis sie bestätigt und schließlich aufgelöst werden. Ihr Ego liebt das Drama, weil es damit vertraut ist und weil es sich bei etwas, das es kennt, sicher fühlt. Es hat stets Angst vor Neuem und möchte nicht loslassen. Es möchte so viel wie möglich die Kontrolle haben.

Schlüssel Nummer fünf:
Uns selbst neu programmieren

Stellen Sie sich vor, Sie begeben sich zum ersten Mal in Ihrem Leben auf eine einsame Insel. Sie fürchten sich ein wenig vor dem, was Ihnen dort bevorstehen wird. Und Sie beschließen, all Ihre alten Glaubenssätze, Muster und Gewohnheiten am Ufer zurückzulassen. Wenn Sie aufbrechen, stellen Sie sich vor, dass Ihr Leben neu beginnt. Der erste Tag eines neuen Lebens. Stellen Sie sich vor, Sie seien völlig frei und unbehindert durch sämtliche menschliche Konzepte. Frei von Angst, Geldmangel etc. Stellen Sie sich vor, Sie seien unschuldig und frei und froh darüber, am Leben zu sein.

Wenn Sie auf der einsamen Insel ankommen, blicken Sie sich um und sehen Sie nach, was Sie finden können. Vielleicht werden Sie nach einem Ort Ausschau halten, der Ihnen Unterschlupf vor der Sonne und dem Regen gewährt. Vielleicht werden Sie eine wunderschöne geöffnete Villa entdecken, die Ihre Ankunft bereits erwartete. Ihr erschafft das, wie Eure neue Zukunft aussehen wird – und das ist Eure Wahrheit, meine Lieben.

Wie auch immer Sie Ihre Zukunft gerne hätten, stellen Sie es sich vor, spüren Sie es, sehen Sie es vor Ihnen, und es wird auf Sie zukommen. Das ist das Gesetz des Lebens, es kann nicht versagen. In jedem Augenblick erschaffen Sie mit Ihren Gedanken, Worten und Taten. Dies ist Ihre Welt, genauso, wie Sie sie haben wollten. Sollten zufälligerweise Dinge in Ihrer Vorstellung auftauchen, die Sie nicht mehr haben möchten, so sagen Sie diesen, sie mögen verschwinden. Sie haben keine Macht über Sie, wenn Sie es nicht zulassen. Sie bekommen das, worauf Sie Ihre Aufmerksamkeit richten.

Wenn Sie sich eine wunderbare, glückliche und wohlhabende Zukunft wünschen, sollten Sie in diesem Augenblick beginnen und dies in Ihrem Geist, mit Ihren Gefühlen und Handlungen erschaffen, indem Sie anordnen: ICH BIN wohlhabend. ICH BIN glücklich, fröhlich und kreativ in jedem Augenblick und lasse nichts anderes als Gottes Vollkommenheit und Liebe in mein Leben eintreten.

Es funktioniert wirklich, meine Lieben. Beginnt bitte in diesem Moment, die Art und Weise zu ändern, wie

Ihr über Euch und andere denkt. Dies ist die einzige Möglichkeit, wie Ihr Euer Leben verändern könnt. Übernehmt die Verantwortung für alles, was Ihr erschaffen habt und wenn Euch das, was Ihr seht, nicht gefällt, solltet Ihr die in Kapitel fünf erwähnten Schritte – Schritte 1-7, durchgehen und von vorne beginnen, jetzt gleich. Es hat keinen Zweck, sich zu beschweren und das Opfer zu spielen. Diese Zeiten sind für immer vorbei und Ihr könnt so frei werden wie ein Vogel am Himmel, indem Ihr die Zukunft erschafft, die Ihr in Eurer Umgebung gerne hättet. Begreift die Weisheit, die mit diesen Worten vermittelt wird, meine Lieben. Wir möchten, dass Ihr alle Eure Freiheit erlangt. Habt Ihr nicht ohnehin schon lange genug gelitten?

Wenn Sie Ihre neue Zukunft angeordnet haben und sich scheinbar nichts verändert, dann ist es zwangsläufig so, dass Sie in gewisser Weise die positiven Affirmationen durch negative Gedankenmuster rückgängig machen. Rufen Sie Ihre mächtige ICH-BIN-Gegenwart an, die in Ihrem Herzen wohnt, um das zu transformieren, was auch immer Sie daran hindert, erfolgreich zu sein. Tun Sie dies solange, bis Sie merken, dass eine Veränderung eingetreten ist. Im Laufe vieler Inkarnationen haben wir viel Geröll angehäuft. Aber machen Sie sich keine Sorgen – wenn Sie aufrichtig das Gesetz der Vergebung anrufen, wird Ihnen sofort vergeben werden. Was für ein Segen!

Kapitel sieben

Schlüssel Nummer sechs: Vergessen Sie alle Begrenzungen

Heute möchten wir mit Euch über das Leben im Allgemeinen sprechen. Wenn das Leben nicht so im Fluss ist, fragen wir uns oft, was schief gelaufen ist. Grundsätzlich wird jedes Baby voller Unschuld und Freiheit geboren. Es ist nur so, dass das Kind durch die Konditionierung seitens der Gesellschaft und Familie und Eltern in vielfacher Hinsicht beschränkt wird. Begrenzungen seitens der Familie machen sich bemerkbar, und das Kind hat Angst davor, nicht alles erreichen zu können, was es möchte. Aufgrund dieser alten Glaubenssysteme, die wir von Gesellschaft, Schule, Familie und Freunden übernommen haben, werden den Kindern diese Begrenzungen auferlegt. Allmählich hat das Kind kein Selbstvertrauen mehr, und sein ursprüngliches Selbstbewusstsein schwindet rasch dahin.

Wie können wir dieses energetische Ungleichgewicht in unseren Familien heutzutage beheben?

Es gibt nur eine Möglichkeit, und diese besteht darin, alles zu vergessen, was Ihnen nicht mehr dienlich ist, und einen Neuanfang zu machen! Begeben Sie sich in Ihrer Vorstellung noch einmal auf diese einsame Insel. Und bevor Sie aufbrechen, lassen Sie bewusst alle alten Glaubenssysteme, Gewohnheiten und Muster los, wie in Kapitel zwei beschrieben. Haben Sie keine Angst vor diesem Vorgang.

Schreiben Sie alle alten Gewohnheiten, Muster, Glaubenssätze auf, die Sie loswerden möchten, und lassen Sie sie nacheinander los. Brechen Sie auf Ihre imaginäre Reise zu der einsamen Insel auf und beginnen Sie, ein neues Leben zu erschaffen, genau so, wie Sie es haben möchten.

Folgen Sie in jedem Augenblick Ihrem Herzen, und Sie werden feststellen, dass sich Ihr ganzes Leben ändern wird. Jeder Tag wird sich auf magische Weise entfalten, wenn Sie dem Gott in Ihnen folgen. Darauf hat die Menschheit vergessen. Ihr habt Gott aus Euch selbst entfernt, obwohl in Wahrheit jeder von Euch ein Teil von Gott ist.

Jeder Mensch, jeder Baum, jede Pflanze und jedes Tier ist ein Teil von Gott. Sie brauchen nur zu akzeptieren, dass Gott in Ihnen lebt und dass Sie ein Teil von Gott sind, der jetzt auf diesem Planeten wandelt. Erlauben Sie es Gott, Ihrem inneren Wissen, Ihrer Intuition, Ihrem Herzen, Sie in jedem Augenblick zu führen.

Wenn Sie dazu angeregt werden, etwas zu tun, was Ihrem Verstand richtig irrational erscheint, sollten Sie es tun, und lassen Sie zu, dass sich die Magie entfaltet. Sie werden erstaunt sein, wie sich Ihr Leben verändern wird. Wenn Sie das innere Gefühl haben, dass ein neues Wagnis nicht ratsam ist, dann tun Sie es nicht! Wenn etwas passiert ist, sagt man oft: „Ich wusste, es wäre besser gewesen, wenn ich dieses oder jenes nicht getan hätte, ich wusste es!" Folgen Sie das nächste Mal Ihrem Herzen, und Ihr Leben wird sich mit viel mehr Leichtigkeit und Anmut entfalten.

Der Gott in Ihnen möchte, dass Sie bei allem, was Sie tun, glücklich, wohlhabend, fröhlich und erfolgreich sind. Er möchte, dass Sie die ganze Zeit über glücklich sind. Allein Ihre negativen Denkmuster und Emotionen verursachen Ihnen Schmerzen. Wenn Sie jeden Gedanken, jedes Wort und jede Tat beobachten, wird die Menschheit viel glücklicher sein. Alles, was Sie aussenden, ob positiv oder negativ, kehrt zu Ihnen zurück, also wenn Sie nur liebevolle Gedanken, Worte und Taten haben, raten Sie mal, was dann zurückkehrt!

Bitten Sie um die Unterstützung der Meister des Lichts, Jesus, Mutter Maria, Saint Germain, bzw. desjenigen, zu wem auch immer Sie sich verbunden fühlen. Sie werden Sie sofort bei Ihren Bemühungen unterstützen, wenn Sie sie darum bitten.

Im Grunde genommen geht es hier darum, sich zu erinnern, wer Sie in Wirklichkeit sind. Sie sind weitaus mehr als nur das menschliche Wesen, das auf dem Planeten um sein Überleben kämpft. Sie sind ein mächtiges Lichtwesen, das auf vielen Ebenen und in vielen Dimensionen existiert. Das Leben in dieser Welt der dritten und vierten Dimension hat dazu geführt, dass Sie vergessen haben, wer Sie in Wirklichkeit sind.

Es ist Zeit, aufzuwachen, meine Lieben, und Euch daran zu erinnern, wer Ihr wirklich seid und dies in Anspruch zu nehmen. Wenn Ihr Eure Wahrheit beansprucht und lebt, werdet Ihr fähig sein, ein großartiges Wesen auf Erden zu werden. Das Leben ist wie ein Spiel, es geht darum, den Himmel auf Erden zu verwirklichen, dass bedeutet, in einer physischen Welt und in einem physischen Körper mit all den Vorteilen, der Schönheit und dem Wissen aus den höheren Reichen zu leben. Es bedeutet, in Freiheit zu leben, und zwar so, wie Ihr von Spirit, Eurem höheren Selbst, Gott, der Intuition, dem Herzen, oder wie immer Ihr es nennen möchtet, geführt werdet!

Kapitel acht

Schlüssel Nummer sieben: Loslassen von allen Ängsten

Ihr durchlebt Zeiten, die von großer Veränderung geprägt sind. Ihr geht von der dritten in die vierte Dimension über, und schließlich in die fünfte und darüber hinaus. Die Realität Eurer Dimension entspricht dem, wo Ihr an diesem Moment steht, mit Euren Gedanken, Worten und Taten. Wenn Ihr Angst habt, lebt Ihr in diesem Moment in der Realität der dritten oder vierten Dimension. Wenn Ihr ständig in Einklang seid und Euer Leben auf liebevolle Weise führt, nähert Ihr Euch der oberen vierten Dimension. Das hängt alles davon ab, wo Ihr in diesem Moment befindet. Mutter Erde wird in die fünfte Dimension aufsteigen, und diejenigen, die diese Realität von bedingungsloser Liebe, Frieden, Freude und Fülle bewahren können, werden an dieser Realität teilhaben können. Das bedeutet, dass wir uns in eine weniger dichte Form der Materie verwandeln werden, die in einer höheren Schwingung lebt. Je mehr wir uns entwickeln, desto weniger dicht sind wir und desto höher wird unsere Schwingung sein! Ihr werdet immer leichter und heller!

In der fünften Dimension hat die Angst keinen Platz mehr. In dieser Zeit ist die gesamte Menschheit auf Erden gezwungen, all ihren Ängsten gegenüberzustehen. Dies ermöglicht es Ihnen, diese Ängste zu spüren und anzusehen. Es gibt jedem die Gelegenheit, herauszufinden, dass diese so genannten Ängste überhaupt keine Macht haben, nur die Macht, die Sie ihnen geben. Ängste sind nur Gefühle (falsche Beweise, die real aussehen!) und sobald Sie Ihre Aufmerksamkeit auf Liebe, Freude, Dankbarkeit, Fülle und Erfolg richten, werden diese Gefühle das Kommando über Ihre Realität und Ihr Leben übernehmen, und sämtliche Ängste werden sich auflösen, da Sie ihnen keine Aufmerksamkeit mehr schenken. Dies ist eine der wichtigsten Lektionen, die die Menschheit zu lernen und zu erinnern hat.

Die Menschen leben in ständiger Angst davor, dass etwas passieren wird. Der einzige Weg, diese Ängste zu überstehen, ist, jeder einzelnen dieser Ängste gegenüberzutreten. Nach dem Sieg, bei dem Sie Ihre Ängste überstanden haben, werden Sie sich sehr ermächtigt fühlen. Es ist eine wirkliche Herausforderung, und Sie werden bei jeder Angst, die Sie überstehen, sehr stolz auf sich sein. In Wahrheit, meine Lieben, gibt es nichts zu fürchten. Es ist nur so, dass Euch Eure alten Glaubenssysteme und Gedankenformen in diese begrenzende Erfahrung und dieses Gefühl der Angst versetzen.

Obwohl es manchmal sehr furchterregend sein kann, wenn man auf seine Gefühle hört, sollten Sie es trotzdem tun. Der erste Gedanke kommt immer von Spirit, und dann schreitet der Verstand ein und versucht, Sie davon abzubringen, dies zu tun, weil ...... Hören Sie auf Ihre Intuition, sie ist immer der beste Führer, und wenn Sie ihr folgen, werden Sie feststellen, dass sich Ihr neues Leben mit Leichtigkeit entfaltet. Praktizieren Sie dies täglich. Bitten Sie Gott, die ICH-BIN-Gegenwart in Ihnen, Sie fortwährend zu führen und zu lehren.

Gott ist der treusorgende Vater, der alle Dinge bereitstellt. Er möchte, dass Ihr Euer Erbe in Anspruch nehmt und zu den großartigen Wesen werdet, die Ihr bereits seid. Ihr seid die Erschaffer Eurer Welten. Entscheidet Euch nun dafür, voller Liebe, Schönheit, Freude, Glückseligkeit, Fülle und Anmut zu erschaffen. Folgt Euren Herzen und macht weisen Gebrauch vom Geschenk des freien Willens.

Kapitel neun

Schlüssel Nummer acht: Die Wahrheit wird Sie befreien

Meine Lieben, diese Zeiten sind für Euch alle nicht leicht. Alles, was nicht hundertprozentig mit der Wahrheit übereinstimmt, wird an die Oberfläche kommen, um es betrachten zu können. Seien Sie sich in jedem Augenblick bewusst, was Sie sagen, denken und tun, denn Sie erschaffen Ihre neue Zukunft. Wenn Ihnen Gedanken oder Worte in den Sinn kommen, die Sie in Ihrer Zukunft nicht mehr haben möchten, lassen Sie diese sofort los. Halten Sie in keinster Weise am Alten fest. Gehen Sie weiter und vertrauen Sie, was Ihre Zukunft anbelangt, auf Gott: „Lass los und überlass es Gott", ist alles, was wir hierzu immer wieder sagen können.

Wagen Sie keine Schritte, es sei denn, diese werden von Ihrem Herzen und Ihrem Geist angeleitet. Reflektieren Sie in jedem Augenblick und fragen Sie sich, was Ihnen Ihr Herz sagt, und folgen Sie den Anweisungen, die Sie unmittelbar erhalten, um weiteren Schmerz und weiteres Leid zu vermeiden. Die Lektionen müssen gelernt werden, und daher werden sie in immer stärkerer Form erscheinen, bis Sie schließlich verstehen, worum es bei der Lektion geht.

Folgen Sie in jedem Augenblick Ihrem Herzen und Ihrem Geist. Handeln Sie nur dann, wenn Sie geführt werden – lassen Sie sich nicht dermaßen einschüchtern, dass Sie voreilige Entscheidungen treffen, weil Sie jemand oder etwas unter Druck setzt. Gott steht niemals unter Zeitdruck. Alles entfaltet sich stets zum göttlichen Zeitpunkt. Wenn jemand versucht, Sie zu einer Entscheidung zu drängen, so ist dies nicht gottgegeben, sondern wurde von der Angst des Egos davor, die Kontrolle über die Situation zu verlieren, hervorgerufen, und in diesem Fall sollten Sie daran denken, dass Spirit nicht auf diese Weise arbeitet. Alles, was Spirit betrifft, entwickelt sich mit Leichtigkeit und Anmut. Dies soll bitte eine Warnung sein, meine Lieben.

Schlüssel Nummer neun: Lassen Sie das Alte los! Lassen Sie los und überlassen Sie es Gott

Nehmt Euch in Acht vor falschen Propheten. In Wahrheit lebe ich im Herzen jedes Mannes, jeder Frau und jedes Kindes. Mein Bewusstsein wächst in jedem von Euch, und mit jedem Schritt, den Ihr auf Eurem spirituellen Weg geht, entfacht dieses Wissen mehr von dieser Weisheit im Inneren, die Ihr dann an andere Leute, wie Freunde oder Nachbarn, weitergeben könnt.

Ihr, diejenigen, die dieses Buch lesen, seid jene, die zugestimmt haben, sich selbst und anderen dabei zu helfen, diese einfachen Wahrheiten zu verstehen. Zuerst, meine Lieben, sollt Ihr die Lektionen selbst lernen, damit Ihr die Weisheit hervorbringen könnt, um anderen zu helfen. Schwierige Zeiten stehen bevor, allerdings betrifft dies nur jene, die das Alte nicht loslassen wollen. Denn für diejenigen, die bereit sind, weiterzugehen, wird die Zukunft von Magie, Schönheit, Freude, Glück und Fülle erfüllt sein. Es wird ein großer Vertrauensvorschuss erforderlich sein – Ihr werdet dazu gezwungen sein, das Alte gänzlich loszulassen, sodass nichts mehr übrig ist, an dem Ihr Euch festhalten könnt. Wir versichern Euch jedoch, dass es sich für Euch lohnen wird.

Wir bitten Euch, jeden Aspekt Eures Lebens zu überprüfen und ganz ehrlich zu Euch selbst zu sein.

Was funktioniert nicht und warum? Meditiert zu diesen Fragen, und die Antworten werden Euch offenbart werden, wenn Ihr darum bittet. Wir bitten Euch in aller Ernsthaftigkeit und Liebe, dies jeden Tag zu tun.

Beginnt, indem Ihr ehrlich und aufrichtig zu Euch selbst seid, in Bezug auf alles, mit dem Ihr in Eurem Leben nicht zufrieden seid, in Bezug auf alle Dinge, die nicht mit Leichtigkeit und Anmut fließen. Fragt Euch selbst, warum? Vielleicht seid Ihr nicht Eurem Geist gefolgt. In den kommenden Zeiten wird nichts funktionieren, wenn Ihr nicht Eurem Herzen folgt. Die Wahrheit soll Euch befreien, und sie wird all jene befreien, die ihre Wahrheit beanspruchen und diese leben. Die anderen werden noch ein wenig länger leiden müssen, bis sie die Lektion gelernt haben, dass sie ihrem Herzen und ihrem Geist folgen sollen, ganz gleich, wie erschreckend dies sein mag. Dies ist der Vertrauensvorschuss, den Ihr nun brauchen werdet. Keinem Menschen auf diesem Planeten wird dies erspart bleiben.

Aus diesem Grund seid Ihr in dieser Zeit inkarniert – um diese wunderbare Gelegenheit zu bekommen, Euch weiter zu entwickeln als in vielen normalen Leben. Wir wissen und verstehen, dass dies nicht leicht ist, denn wir haben Euch den Weg geebnet, damit Ihr in unsere Fußstapfen treten könnt. Wir mussten jede Lektion lernen, die Ihr nun lernt. Wir sind immer bei Euch und warten nur darauf, dass wir von Euch um

Hilfe gebeten werden. Bittet und es soll Euch gegeben werden.

Geht weiter voller Vertrauen, und Eure Zukunft wird Schritt für Schritt offenbart werden. Nichts ist in diesen kommenden Zeiten vorhersagbar. Alles wird innerhalb des göttlichen Planes verändert und neu gestaltet werden. Habt keine Angst, meine Lieben.

Wir wissen, dass Euer Verstand sein Spiel mit Euch treibt und versucht, Eure Herzen davon zu überzeugen, dass etwas nicht stimmt, da scheinbar nichts mehr so funktioniert, wie dies einst war. Schenkt diesem Drama keinen Glauben, denn es entspricht nicht der Wahrheit. Es ist nur so, dass sich alles ändert und dass nichts mehr vertraut ist. Um in diesen Zeiten großer Veränderung zu überleben, werdet Ihr eine Menge an Vertrauen brauchen, denn viele werden sich von Katastrophen mitreißen lassen, und allein schon die Atmosphäre, in der Ihr lebt, wird ansteckend sein.

Die einzige Möglichkeit, wie Ihr Euch davon fernhalten könnt, ist, täglich zu meditieren. Ladet Euch selbst wieder mit der Energie des Schöpfers auf. Geht so viel wie möglich in die Natur und reinigt Euch selbst in Flüssen, in Teichen und im Ozean. Es wäre auch hilfreich, als Reinigungsritual Dusch- und Vollbäder zu nehmen. Je mehr Ihr bewusst etwas tut, desto besser.

Viele von Euch fragen sich: „Warum sind wir hier, was sollen wir tun?" Viele von Euch haben wenig Selbstvertrauen, weil scheinbar nichts mehr so funktioniert wie einst. Das ist auch nicht möglich. Es hat nichts mit Euch persönlich zu tun – mit Euren Talenten oder der Art und Weise, wie Ihr arbeitet. Es hat etwas mit dem Anbruch des goldenen Zeitalters zu tun. Das Alte zerfällt täglich, und das Neue ist noch nicht angekommen. Es sieht buchstäblich so aus, als würde Eure ganze Welt rund um Euch zerbröckeln, und dies ist eine Tatsache. Ihr seid nicht die Einzigen, dies geschieht überall und mit jedem. Manche werden den Prozess vor den anderen durchmachen, damit sie ihnen später helfen können.

Ihr könnt diesen Prozess nicht aufhalten, meine Lieben, und daher bitten wir Euch, Eure Versuche, dies zu bekämpfen und sich dagegen zu wehren, zu beenden. Akzeptiert, dass sich die Welt rapide verändert und dass weder Ihr noch jemand anderer etwas tun kann, um es aufzuhalten. Akzeptiert jeden Tag als eine neue Herausforderung und fragt Euch selbst: „Was wird sich heute ereignen?" Seht den ganzen Vorgang als ein Abenteuer und hört ein für alle Mal auf, Euch als Opfer dieses Vorgangs zu fühlen.

Ihr habt Euch dafür entschieden, hier zu sein. Macht nun weiter und hört auf, Euch selbst zu bemitleiden! Es ist höchste Zeit für Euch, dass Ihr die Zukunft fortsetzt und aufhört, einer Vergangenheit nachzuweinen, die nicht mehr wirksam ist. Wir wissen und verstehen, dass es nicht leicht für Euch ist, weil Ihr kein Vorbild habt, dem Ihr folgen könnt. Ihr seid die Vorreiter, die Wegweiser, die dem Rest der Menschheit den Weg ebnen und die den anderen nur ein kleines Bisschen voraus sind!

Seid in jedem Augenblick im Frieden und lasst nicht zu, dass Euch andere mit ihren Gefühlen und Launen beeinflussen. Wir sprechen jedem Einzelnen von Euch Dank und Anerkennung dafür aus, dass Ihr Euch traut, die Vorreiter zu sein. Wir wissen, dass es nicht leicht ist, doch die Belohnung wird großartig sein.

Dieser Zeitraum des Übergangs zwischen den Welten wird ungefähr fünf Jahre dauern. Dies mag Euch sehr lange vorkommen, wenn Ihr Angst habt, doch in Wahrheit wird es lange genug dauern, sodass die gesamte Menschheit aufholen kann. Die meisten werden überhaupt keine Ahnung von den bevorstehenden Veränderungen haben, und diejenigen von Euch, die verstehen, was nun geschieht, werden sie darüber informieren müssen. Sie werden viel Unterstützung und Ermutigung brauchen, wenn die Dinge schwierig werden. Es wird den Anschein haben, als hätte Gott die Menschheit verlassen, weil es viel zu bewältigen geben wird. In Wahrheit wird es Euch aber die Gelegenheit geben, alle Themen in Eurem Leben anzusehen, die Eurer Aufmerksamkeit oder einer Veränderung bedürfen. Kein einziger Mensch wird davon verschont werden. Viele werden sich dazu entschließen, zu gehen, weil die Schmerzen einfach zu groß sein werden. Diejenigen von Euch, die den Mut haben, weiterzugehen und sich alles anzusehen, dass angesehen werden muss, um Euch das Weitergehen zu ermöglichen, werden eine helle und glorreiche Zukunft vor sich haben – eine Realität, die auf dem Planeten Erde noch nie erlebt wurde. Also wartet noch und genießt es. Der Schlüssel liegt darin, Augenblick für Augenblick im JETZT zu leben.

Meine Geliebten, wir danken jedem von Euch für Eure aufrichtigen Bemühungen bei Eurem Streben nach Vollkommenheit. Oftmals erzeugt das Streben nach Meisterschaft und Vollkommenheit eine Blockade, weil Ihr so auf ein konkretes Ziel konzentriert seid, dass Euch die Magie des „Jetzt" entgeht. Wir möchten Euch wissen lassen, meine Lieben, dass Ihr alle aus eigener Kraft Meister seid – jeder Einzelne von Euch. Konzentriert Euch darauf, anstatt Euch auf den Mangel zu konzentrieren.

Die Illusion der irdischen Ebene und der Vergesslichkeit, die Ihr betreten habt, ist sehr real, wenn Ihr im Zentrum des Dramas gefangen seid. Sobald Ihr es von unserem Blickwinkel, vom größeren Bild aus, betrachtet, werdet Ihr erkennen, dass es nichts gibt, worüber Ihr bestürzt sein müsst, da alles eine Illusion ist.

Es ist nur ein Spiel, das Ihr in der Realität der dritten und vierten Dimension ausspielt, während Ihr Euch abmüht und alles sehr ernst nehmt.

Ärgert Euch nicht mehr, meine Geliebten. Es ist nun an der Zeit, zu erkennen, wer Ihr in Wirklichkeit seid, und das kleine Bild zu vergessen. Seid Euch bewusst, dass Ihr weitaus mehr seid, als Ihr Euch vorstellen könnt. Das große Bild ist riesig, und jeder von Euch ist ein kosmisches Wesen mit einem großen Wissen. Nur ein kleiner Bruchteil Eurer Seele willigte ein, noch einmal zu inkarnieren, in dem Versuch, das Spiel diesmal richtig zu spielen. Verbessert das Ergebnis.

Es ist alles ein Spiel. Sobald Ihr dies zu verstehen beginnt, werdet Ihr das Leben und Euch selbst nicht so ernst nehmen. Genießt jeden Tag in vollen Zügen; lebt im Jetzt; strebt nicht nach Dingen, die Ihr nicht habt. Diese Erkenntnis macht einen Bruchteil davon aus, wer Ihr seid, und das höhere Selbst weiß alles! Es ist so, als würde man Blindekuh spielen!

Nehmt nicht alles so tragisch. Lebt jeden Tag und nehmt jeden Moment als einen Teil der Rolle an, die Ihr spielt, und seht zu, wie sich das Magische entwickeln wird. Lasst nicht zu, dass das Drama der äußeren Welt – von Menschen erschaffenes Desaster und Angst – Eure Reinheit befleckt. Schenkt keiner dieser Geschichten Glauben.

Worauf auch immer Ihr Euch konzentriert, genau das werdet Ihr in Eurem Leben anziehen. Seid in jedem Augenblick in Frieden und genießt die prächtige Schönheit von Mutter Erde, die hier ist, damit sich alle an ihr erfreuen können. Je mehr Ihr Euch auf Katastrophen und Probleme konzentriert, desto eher werdet Ihr dies erleben. Je mehr Ihr Euch auf Freude, Friede, Glück und Fülle konzentriert, desto eher werdet Ihr dies in Eurer Welt erleben.

In Wahrheit lebt jeder Mensch in jedem Augenblick seine oder ihre Realität. Es gibt nicht nur eine Realität. Jeder Mensch auf diesem Planeten und jenseits davon erschafft in jedem Augenblick seine eigene Lebenserfahrung.

Begreift die Weisheit dieser Worte, meine Lieben. Wir möchten, dass Ihr alle Eure Freiheit erlangt.

Wenn Sie Ihre neue Zukunft angeordnet haben und sich scheinbar nichts verändert, dann ist es zwangsläufig so, dass Sie in gewisser Weise die positiven Affirmationen durch negative Gedankenmuster rückgängig machen. Rufen Sie Ihre mächtige ICH-BIN-Gegenwart an, um sämtliche Blockaden in Ihrem Geist, Ihrem Körper und Ihrer Welt zu transformieren und zu beseitigen. Rufen Sie die Unterstützung des geliebten Erzengels Michael und seiner Legionen von Engeln herbei, um mit dem blauen Blitz von zehntausend Sonnen zu erscheinen und sämtliche schädliche Energie zu verbrennen. Bitten Sie ihn, Sie zu befreien und von der gesamten menschlichen Schöpfung freizumachen und alles in der mächtigen violetten Flamme zu transformieren. Ordnen Sie dies solange an, bis Sie eine Veränderung der Energie wahrnehmen.

Diese tägliche Anordnung ist ein sehr kraftvolles Werkzeug. Fühlen Sie es, sehen Sie es und seien Sie sich bewusst, dass es geschehen wird, auch wenn es noch nicht manifestiert wurde. Dies ist das Gesetz des Universums.

Diese Botschaft ist von großer Bedeutung, meine Lieben, und hiermit möchten wir Teil I beenden. Es folgt das Kapitel zehn, welches von Sue verfasst wurde, um uns an einer persönlichen Erfahrung teilhaben zu lassen.

Teil II

Kapitel zehn

Die Seele

Soweit ich aus meiner eigenen Erfahrung berichten kann, steigt unser höheres Selbst in unseren physischen Körper hinab, während wir alte Muster und Emotionen in unseren vier niedrigeren Körpern reinigen und säubern. Jedes Mal, wenn wir das Alte loslassen und dadurch geheilt und einheitlich werden, erhöhen wir die Schwingung unseres Körpers, sodass wir mehr Licht aufnehmen können. Dieser Prozess wirkt sich auf Mutter Erde aus, und wie Sie wahrscheinlich schon bemerkt haben, beschleunigt sich die Zeit, während sich das Licht ausdehnt. Auch die Mutter Erde bewegt sich in Richtung Aufstieg. Dies bedeutet, dass wir als Ganzes auf eine andere Dimension zusteuern. Wir selbst gehen nirgendwohin, sondern in Wirklichkeit handelt es sich hierbei um ein Hinabsteigen des Geistes in die Materie, die nicht mehr so dicht sein wird, wie dies in der Vergangenheit der Fall war. Dies ist ein allmählicher Prozess, der jahrelange sorgfältige Selbsterkenntnis in Verbindung mit einer Menge an Loslösungsarbeit erfordert, was aber nicht mehr anstrengend sein muss! Wenn wir bereit sind, unsere irdischen Agenden loszulassen, steigt die mächtige ICH-BIN-Gegenwart Schritt für Schritt hinunter in unsere physischen Körper. Langsam, aber sicher übernimmt der höhere Aspekt des Selbst, der in anderen Dimensionen und Realitäten verweilt, das Kommando. Damit dies geschehen kann, müssen wir alles in unserem Leben an unser höchstes Ziel übergeben. Unser Ego muss alles loswerden, wie wir es kennen! Alte Lebens- und Denkweisen, die uns nicht mehr dienlich sind. Die Dinge, die am dringendsten losgelassen werden müssen, sind Schuld, Schmerz, Leid, Opferdasein und die Unfähigkeit zu vergeben, damit wir ein neues Leben voller Freude, Glück, bedingungsloser Liebe, Frieden, harmonischen Beziehungen und Fülle in allen Formen annehmen können.

Wenn dies geschieht, beginnt sich unser gesamtes Leben zu ändern. Wenn wir mehr und mehr an unser göttliches Selbst im Inneren übergeben, werden wir erfüllt von einem sich stetig erweiternden, Licht, bedingungsloser Liebe und Mitgefühl. Wir werden uns allmählich für jede kleine Sache in unserem Leben äußerst dankbar, gesegnet und glücklich fühlen. Dies ist wahrhaftig eine wunderbare und aufregende Reise, und sie ist die Schwierigkeiten, denen wir entlang des Weges begegnen, sehr wohl wert!

Ich werde Ihnen nun meine persönliche Geschichte erzählen, damit dieser Prozess jenen von Ihnen, die ihn vielleicht in ähnlicher Weise durchmachen werden, nicht so viel Angst einflößen wird und damit Sie etwas haben, worauf Sie sich beziehen können. Seien Sie sich bewusst, dass alles in göttlicher Ordnung ist und dass alles einen Teil des göttlichen Planes für die Menschheit zu dieser Zeit darstellt.

Dieser allmähliche Prozess hatte plötzlich seinen Höhepunkt erreicht, und es erweckte den Anschein, als würde sich alles auflösen! Alles, was mir und meiner Familie nicht mehr von Nutzen war, brach zusammen. Es sah wirklich so aus, als könnte es nicht mehr dunkler werden! Jeder von uns, der bereit ist, sich zu verändern und spirituell zu wachsen, wird diesen Prozess in der einen oder anderen Art früher oder später durchmachen müssen. Dieser Prozess wird als die dunkle Nacht der Seele bezeichnet.

Im März 2000 übersiedelten wir in ein wunderschönes altes Haus am Strand von Maui. Mein Traum war in Erfüllung gegangen, denn ich wollte schon immer am Strand oder neben dem Strand leben. Ich war so dankbar und glücklich darüber, dass dies wahr geworden war. Ich hatte diesen Traum tatsächlich manifestiert, indem ich mir vorgestellt hatte, wie es sich anfühlen würde, jeden Tag mit Honey, unserem Golden Retriever, am Strand entlang zu spazieren und zu schwimmen. Die Einzelheiten unseres Hauses waren praktisch identisch mit meiner Wunschliste! Ich hatte es nicht nur geschafft, ein Leben auf Maui zu manifestieren, sondern auch das perfekte, dazugehörige Haus. Ich befand mich in einem Zustand vollkommener Glückseligkeit!

Während das Leben seinen Fortlauf nahm und das Unternehmen meines Mannes Harry scheinbar nicht anlaufen wollte, hatte ich diese immer wiederkehrende Angst, dass es uns vielleicht nicht gelingen würde, unseren Traum zu bewahren. Tief im Inneren wusste ich, dass ich vertrauen musste und nicht mehr zulassen durfte, dass die Angst meinen Traum ergriff. Ich war der Schöpfer meiner Realität und musste mich auf das konzentrieren, was ich erschaffen wollte, denn ich wusste, wie das Ergebnis aussehen würde, wenn ich das nicht tat! Wir führten ein glückliches Leben, allerdings in großer Unsicherheit, was oft die Freude und Dankbarkeit, die ich für diese wunderbare Gelegenheit, die wir bekommen hatten, verspürte, überschattete. Im Inneren wusste ich, dass ich diese Überlebensangst überwinden musste, denn dies war das Hauptthema, das hier auf dem Spiel stand. Ich wollte dies unbedingt schaffen, denn viele Leute, die auf Maui lebten, lebten in einem Bewusstsein des Mangels. Dies stand natürlich im Widerspruch zu der Wahrheit, die uns allen bekannt war, denn das Universum besteht aus einer grenzenlosen Fülle! Ich hatte es hier mit einem Grundthema zu tun und spürte, dass es an der Zeit war, diese ständig quälende Angst im Hinterkopf zu überwinden! Diese Angst erfasste nicht nur meinen Geist, sondern auch mein gesamter Körper verfiel jedes Mal, wenn mich diese Angst ergriff, in einen toxischen Schock. Ich musste dieses Muster irgendwie überwinden und betete täglich um eine Anleitung dazu, wie ich dies tun könnte. Ich fand heraus, dass das Gehen und Schwimmen mir half, die Energie in meinem Körper zu verlagern. Es erwies sich für mich beruhigend, mich selbst zu lieben, die Angst zu akzeptieren, die Emotionen einzuatmen, die mit der ganzen Erfahrung einhergingen, und mit einem Freund über meine Gefühle zu sprechen.

Es war für mich extrem hilfreich, nach Europa und England zu reisen, Workshops zu veranstalten und private Sitzungen durchzuführen, da ich tatsächlich etwas tat, um unsere Situation zu verbessern. Es war ein gutes Gefühl, aktiv zu sein, zu unterrichten, anderen zu helfen und wieder Geld zu verdienen! Ich erlangte mein Selbstvertrauen wieder und beanspruchte meine Macht, und das fühlte sich wunderbar an! Ich kehrte erschöpft, aber glücklich zurück und hatte das Gefühl, es sei zu viel für mich, allein die Verantwortung für den Erhalt der Familie zu haben, und es war Zeit, dass auch mein Mann wieder mit einer Tätigkeit begann! Von diesem Moment an entspannte ich mich und hoffte, dass er sich an die Arbeit machen würde. Eine Gruppe mit sechzehn Leuten aus Europa kam zu uns, und wir boten gemeinsam Inselrundfahrten zu den heiligen Plätzen an, und das war eine ganz wunderbare Sache. Nachdem sie uns verlassen hatten, wusste ich, dass nichts mehr so sein würde wie früher und die Zukunft erschien trostlos und sehr düster. Ich sah die Zukunft näher rückten, alles war leer!

Einige Wochen später kehrte ich von meinem täglichen Spaziergang und meiner Schwimmrunde zurück und wurde von Harry begrüßt, der mir einen Brief von einem Fachanwalt der Einwanderungsbehörde entgegenhielt, in dem geschrieben stand, dass unser Visum nicht verlängert worden war und dass uns noch neunzig Tage blieben, um zu entscheiden, was wir tun wollten! Die ganze Familie war am Boden zerstört und bestürzt.

Was sollen wir jetzt tun, und wohin sollten wir gehen? Wir hatten bereits einmal unseren ganzen Besitz aufgegeben, um nach Maui zu kommen, und nun wurden wir wiederum gebeten, alles aufzugeben. Es schien einfach nicht fair zu sein. Ich weinte tagelang, konnte nicht mehr klar denken und fühlte mich wie ein Opfer! Warum tat Gott uns das an, fragte ich mich selbst dauernd, was hatte ich getan, um so eine Behandlung zu verdienen? Wir hatten stets andere unterstützt, die vom Glück nicht so begünstigt waren, und hatten geholfen, wo wir konnten! Ich war erfüllt von Zorn und Kummer, stapfte jeden Morgen den Strand hinauf und hinunter und setzte all diese Gefühle frei, die von meinem Inneren ausgingen. Insgeheim wusste ich natürlich, dass wir nicht von Gott bestraft wurden, sondern dass tief im Inneren etwas existierte, das bewirkte, dass ich mich als Opfer dieser ganzen Situation fühlte, weil ich mir so hilflos vorkam. Abgesehen davon hatten wir nur wenig Geld übrig. Harry wollte, dass ich etwas mehr Geld von England überweisen würde, doch ich weigerte mich, denn wir mussten dieses Problem auf eine andere Weise lösen! Das Ironische daran war, dass ich mir über das Geld überhaupt keine Sorgen mehr machte, ich war nur traurig darüber, dass ich mein geliebtes Maui und das Zuhause, das ich so von Herzen liebte, verlassen musste. Ich wusste, dass wir genügend Geld haben würden, um unsere Tickets nach Europa zu erstehen, wenn wir einen Teil unseres Mobiliars, ein Auto und persönliche Sachen verkaufen würden. Es ging nicht mehr um das Überleben, das Thema hatte nun eine andere Ebene erreicht. Ich wusste, dass es uns wunderbar gehen würde, aber ich hatte keine Vorstellung davon, wie!

In der Zwischenzeit entschlossen sich unsere älteste Tochter Melanie und ihr Freund Ben zu heiraten, sie sollten von diesem Drama nicht entzweigerissen werden. Dies schien der nächste Schritt zu sein, und daher begannen wir mit der Planung ihrer Hochzeit, obwohl wir nicht viel Geld dafür hatten. Es stellte sich heraus, dass wie immer alles auf göttliche Weise bereitgestellt wurde und dass wir dank einer Menge an Hilfe von unseren Familien, Bens Familie und Freunden in der Lage waren, ihnen eine wunderschöne Hochzeit in der Nähe des Ozeans zu ermöglichen. Ein Hawaiianer war gekommen, um die Trompetenschnecke (Anm.d. Ü.: große spiralige Meeresschnecke, wird als Trompete verwendet) zu blasen und hawaiianische Musik zu spielen. Währenddessen gab uns ein lieber Freund, ein Schüler des hawaiianischen Kahuna, in hawaiianischer Sprache den Segen. Mirra Rose traute die beiden unter dem führenden Licht des geliebten Christus und der Mutter Maria. Terry, ein weiterer Freund, der über die Gabe des Hellsehens verfügt, sagte uns, dass Christus hinter den beiden stand und sie in seinen Armen hielt und dass Mutter Maria in einem großen Lichtstrahl heruntergekommen war und die beiden vereint hatte. Dies war wahrhaftig eine Ehe, die im Himmel vollzogen wurde. Der Hochzeitsempfang fand in einem Park oberhalb des Strandes statt. Wir hatten eine Menge Spaß zusammen. Es gab ein ausgezeichnetes Buffet, bei dessen Vorbereitung Cherie, die Mutter von Ben, ich selbst und andere Freunde mitgeholfen hatten. Gegen Ende der Hochzeit gingen wir alle schwimmen und sangen gemeinsam Lieder. Dies war bestimmt ein Teil des göttlichen Planes, da alles so mit Leichtigkeit und Anmut dahinfloss.

Wir veranstalteten drei Garagenflohmärkte (Anm. d. Ü.: in einer Garage durchgeführter Verkauf von Haushaltsgegenständen und Trödel), verkauften eines unserer Autos und verschenkten einen Großteil unserer Möbel an Melanie und Ben für ihr neues Zuhause. Sie fanden ein wundervolles neues Landhaus in Kula, das perfekte kleine Liebesnest. Sie zogen Ende November – wenige Tage nach der Hochzeit – dort ein, es war der zweite Ort, den sie besichtigt hatten und er war perfekt!

Eines Tages kam Harry mit drei Flugtickets für Alexander, Serena und mich nach Hause, damit wir am 10. Dezember 2001 zurückfliegen konnten. Ich konnte das nicht ertragen, alles in mir schrie auf, dass ich noch nicht bereit war, Maui zu verlassen. Ich brauchte mehr Zeit, um das, was gerade geschehen war, aufzunehmen.

Alle waren sich einig, dass ich mir einen Tag frei nehmen sollte, um mich von dem Packen und Putzen zu erholen. Ich war gereizt, und ich fühlte mich extrem traurig und vollkommen erschöpft, in geistiger, emotionaler und physischer Hinsicht. Ich machte mich auf, um mit Mirra den Tag am Strand zu verbringen, die mir ein paar gute Ratschläge gab. Sie sagte: „Akzeptiere einfach alles, bewerte es nicht und versuche nicht, die Situation zu verändern, akzeptiere alles, wie es jetzt in diesem Moment ist." Das tat ich auch, und in nur wenigen Stunden am Strand gelang es mir, zu Gott zu sprechen und zu sagte, „Wenn Du wirklich möchtest, dass wir in wenigen Tagen gehen sollen, werden wir das machen, ich übergebe meine Zukunft und die Zukunft meiner Familie an Dich, Gott, denn Du weißt, was für uns alle das Beste ist, Du hast das größere Bild, bitte gib mir ein Zeichen." Ich ließ alles los und ging schwimmen, genoss den Tag und erholte mich von einer erschöpfenden Woche des Packens.

Innerhalb von wenigen Stunden wurde mir sehr klar, dass wir unmöglich weggehen konnten, da wir warten mussten, bis Serena, unsere jüngste Tochter, ihr Highschool-Jahr abgeschlossen hatte. Ihr würde es extreme Schwierigkeiten bereiten, wenn wir während dem Schuljahr in eine andere Schule, ein anderes Land umziehen würden. Plötzlich hatte ich eine Idee, wie wir dies machen konnten! Allmählich sahen die Dinge wieder etwas rosiger aus! Ich ging nach Hause und berichtete Harry von meinem Plan. Ich wollte eine Freundin, die ein Retreat-Zentrum in Huelo besaß, fragen, ob es möglich wäre, dass wir gegen Arbeit im Zentrum wohnen könnt. Auf diese Weise würden wir nicht so viel Geld brauchen und könnten möglicherweise bleiben, wenn man unser Visa verlängern würde! Zu unserem großen Erstaunen erschien wenige Stunden später jene besagte Freundin vor unserer Haustür und sagte, dass ihr Auto in unsere Zufahrt gefahren war und dass sie vorbeikommen musste. Wir stellten die entscheidende Frage und sie willigte ein. Ich kann Ihnen nicht sagen, wie glücklich ich war, dass wir nicht am 10. Dezember 2001 weggehen mussten. Was für eine göttliche Intervention! Ich danke Dir, Gott!

Während dieser ganzen Zeit ging es in dieser Lektion, die wir lernten, um das Leben im hier und JETZT! Jeden Tag änderten sich unsere Pläne, und wir sagten: „Nun, heute sieht es so aus, als würden wir dieses und jenes tun." Es zeigte uns, dass wir unser Leben, nicht in der Hand hatten. Göttliche Kräfte waren im Spiel und wir waren nur die Figuren auf diesem Schachbrett! Ein paar Tage später erhielt Harry ein Angebot, einem Freund in den nächsten drei bis sechs Monaten das Golfspielen beizubringen. Er beschloss, diese wunderbare Gelegenheit anzunehmen, da es ihm etwas mehr Zeit geben würde, um seine Pläne für die Zukunft zu schmieden. Er brauchte nun einen Ort, an dem er leben konnte. Ein anderer Freund hatte zufällig ein kleines Häuschen zu vermieten, und so konnte er am 5. Dezember 2001 einziehen. Es war unglaublich, wie alles floss und wie die Teile des Puzzles Sinn ergaben und wie viele Möbelstücke, die nicht verkauft oder an Melanie und Ben verschenkt worden waren, perfekt in dieses kleine Häuschen passten. Gott hatte hier bestimmt einen Plan, doch wir wussten nichts davon.

Und dieser konnte erst dann ins Spiel kommen, wenn ich alles losgelassen und akzeptiert hatte.

Wenige Tage danach zogen Serena und Harry in dieses kleine Häuschen, und ich ging für einige Monate allein nach Huelo, da ich mich verpflichtet hatte, gegen Arbeit dort zu wohnen. Während mich Alexander, mein Sohn, mit all meinen Habseligkeiten zum Retreat-Zentrum fuhr, fühlte ich mich so, als würde ich noch einmal ins Internat gehen. Hier war ich allein in einem eigenartigen Haus, mitten im Dschungel ohne meine Familie. Ich fühlte mich zuerst sehr einsam, gewöhnte mich aber bald an das Leben in diesem Zentrum. Alle waren sehr freundlich und gaben mir das Gefühl, willkommen zu sein. Als ich eine oder zwei Wochen dort war, blätterte ich mein Tagebuch durch und stieß auf ein Gelübde, das ich an Gott abgelegt hatte, und in dem ich alles übergeben wollte, was ich hatte, weil ich wirklich mit dem Göttlichen eins sein und mit ihm Zwiesprache halten wollte. Plötzlich erinnerte ich mich und verstand, was soeben mit unserem Leben geschehen war. Ich hatte alles übergeben, und als der göttliche Plan ins Spiel kam, hatte ich mein Gelübde ganz vergessen. Plötzlich war alles kristallklar!

Alexander verließ Maui, flog am 10. Dezember nach Österreich und fand eine Arbeitsstelle in einem Skiort bei St. Johann in Tirol. Er lebt nun in Kitzbühel, arbeitet in einem sehr guten Restaurant und liebt diese

Arbeit. (Bei dieser ganzen Angelegenheit hat auch er eine Menge gelernt, und so kann ich ihn und Harry besuchen, wenn ich eine Österreichreise mache. Wir haben ein liebevolles und warmherziges Verhältnis zueinander und freuen uns immer, wenn wir uns wiedersehen.)

Es war eine herausfordernde, aber glückliche Zeit, ganz anders als das Leben, das ich einst gewohnt war. Ich verspürte nur sehr wenige Emotionen, als ob ich mich in einer Leere befände. Ich hatte keine Wünsche oder Ziele für die Zukunft, ich lebte nur von Augenblick zu Augenblick im hier und JETZT. Und das war natürlich genau das, was ich eigentlich tun sollte! Es war auch keine Freude vorhanden, und das war das seltsamste Gefühl überhaupt, weil ich im Allgemeinen ein sehr fröhlicher und glücklicher Mensch bin. Ich fühlte mich völlig anders, als wäre ein Teil von mir während diesem dramatischen Prozess, bei dem unsere Familie so plötzlich entzweigerissen wurde, gestorben. Ich liebte es, eine Mutter zu sein, und schätzte mein Zuhause sehr.

Ich war sehr introvertiert und verbrachte viel Zeit damit, nach innen zu schauen! Ich kämpfte ständig gegen den Impuls, vor dieser ganzen Situation zu flüchten und Serena und Harry in Kihei Gesellschaft zu leisten. Manchmal musste ich mich dazu zwingen, in diesem Zentrum zu bleiben, anstatt sie an meinen freien Tagen zu besuchen. Ich vermisste den Strand und das wunderbare Wetter. Im Dschungel regnete es viel, und manchmal fühlte ich mich richtig wie eine Gefangene, da ich kein Auto hatte und nur dann wegkommen konnte, wenn mich jemand im Auto mitnahm.

Es war sehr demütigend, in einer Position zu sein, bei der ich alles verloren hatte und mir meinen Lebensunterhalt mit dem Putzen verdienen musste. Manchmal kam ich mir wie eine Sklavin vor, was natürlich kein allzu gutes Gefühl war, wie Sie sich vielleicht vorstellen können. Ich wusste, dass ich bis zum Ende durchhalten musste, weil ich einige wunderbare Lektionen lernte. Ich hatte Spaß an der Gartenarbeit und konnte der Mutter auf eine wundervolle Weise dienen. Was das Putzen anging, so konnte ich dabei das Gefühl nicht loswerden, dass ich nichts wert war, wenn ich für jemand anderen putzte. Ich wusste, dass dies eine meiner Lektionen war, und das Einzige, was ich zu tun hatte, war, mich selbst nicht mehr zu beurteilen und mit Freude Gott zu dienen, ohne mich wertlos zu fühlen. Im Geiste wusste ich, dass das, was ich in Wirklichkeit bin, sich nicht durch das verändert wird, was ich tat, wo ich mich aufhielt oder was ich besaß. Der übrige Teil meines Wesens konnte dies scheinbar nicht verstehen.

Eines Tages änderte sich das alles, und ich verstand, dass ich Gott diente, unabhängig davon, was ich tat, und das Putzen veränderte die Tatsache, wer ich war, nicht wirklich! Ich begriff, dass Gott mich genau an dem Ort, an dem ich mich befand, haben wollte. Ich wusste, dass ich meine Gaben und mein Licht mit dem Land und den Menschen in der Umgebung teilte. Von diesem Tag an hatte ich wirklich Spaß. Ich begann, mich selbst wieder zu lieben, und verstand, dass all dies ein Teil des göttlichen Planes war. Ich lernte so viel, während ich dieses schöne Zentrum mit anderen teilte, und überwand dabei viele alte Muster.

Die Seele meiner Mutter erschien mir immer wieder in Visionen, sie rief mich immer wieder zu sich nach Hause, und so verließ ich Huelo Ende Februar, weil ich das Gefühl hatte, dass meine Mission mehr oder weniger erfüllt war. Es gab noch etwas, worauf ich gewartet hatte, ein Versprechen von Spirit, das sich noch nicht manifestiert hatte. Es gab also einen Teil von mir, der immer noch das Gefühl hatte, dass ich in gewisser Hinsicht versagt hätte. Mein Ziel war es, all das Geschwätz in meinem Verstand zu zerstreuen, sodass mir Mutter Maria erscheinen könnte. Ich hatte eine Vision, bei der sie am Horizont aufgetaucht war, aber leider war sie mir zu meiner großen Enttäuschung bis zum Zeitpunkt, an dem ich wegging, nicht erschienen, obwohl ich sie täglich anrief und betete. Ich wusste, dass der Moment gekommen war, an dem ich nach Kihei gehen und Zeit mit Serena, meiner jüngsten Tochter, verbringen sollte, bevor ich nach England zurückkehren würde.

Die nächsten Wochen vergingen schnell, und ich verspürte dieses wunderbare Gefühl von Freude, Frieden, Liebe und Dankbarkeit für mein Leben. Ich war dankbar für jede kleine Angelegenheit. Endlich war ich von der Leere hinaus in das Licht gelangt, und welch ein wunderbares Gefühl es doch war, zu Hause zu sein! Ich lebte mehrere Monate mit Harry und Serena in dem kleinen Landhaus, wo es zwar etwas eng war, aber wir schafften es.

Im März 2002 besuchte ich mit meinen lieben Freunden Colleen Marshall und Sheldan Nidle das Wesak-Festival. Ich half bei ihrem Stand aus und stellte BioGenesis aus, eine heilende Technologie aus der Zeit von Atlantis und ein großes Geschenk an die Menschheit dieser Zeit. (Ich verwende die BioGenesis-Instrumente in meinen Sitzungen und bringe den Leuten bei, wie sie zu gebrauchen sind.) Sheldan war einer der Hauptvortragenden, er war der beste, jeder liebte seine Botschaft, und es wurde noch ein Abendtermin festgelegt, damit er nochmals einen Vortrag halten konnte. Es war ein weiterer inspirierender Abend in Mount Shasta. Dies galt vor allem für mich, denn zu meinem großen Erstaunen erschien mir an diesem Abend Mutter Maria. Es war die wundervollste Erfahrung meines ganzen Lebens. Sie zeigte mir, wie sich göttliche Liebe anfühlte. Es war wirklich ein Geschenk des Göttlichen, und ich werde ewig für diese unvergessliche Erfahrung, die mein Leben veränderte, dankbar sein. Die Liebe strömte wie ein Wasserfall durch mich hindurch. Ich weiß nun, wie sich göttliche Liebe anfühlt, und meine Absicht besteht darin, diesen Zustand die ganze Zeit über aufrechtzuerhalten. Während dieser Zeit fühlte ich mich, als könnte ich so viel Liebe teilen und die Menschen in meiner Umgebung positiv beeinflussen. Was für ein Geschenk!

Als wir wieder in Maui waren, wurde ich mir der sehr deutlichen Botschaft bewusst, dass sich Harry und ich scheiden lassen mussten. Seit wir das Haus am Strand verlassen hatten, war unsere Beziehung nicht mehr wie früher, und wir hatten uns seit vielen Jahren auseinander gelebt. Es war nun Zeit, uns voneinander zu lösen und getrennte Wege zu gehen. Wir wurden ziemlich rasch, im Stillen und friedlich voneinander geschieden, da wir nicht wollten, dass die Kinder und alle Beteiligten zu sehr darunter litten. Wir bekämpften uns nie und stritten auch nie um etwas, es war einfach an der Zeit für uns, eigene Wege zu gehen. Die ganze Situation war für alle sehr traurig. Wir trennten uns, obwohl wir uns noch liebten und wussten, dass jeder von uns weitergehen musste und seine Freiheit brauchte. (Bis heute sind wir ständig in Verbindung und haben eine ausgesprochen liebevolle und glückliche Beziehung zueinander, wofür ich sehr dankbar bin.) Serena und ich gingen dann nach Haiku, wo wir uns ein schönes Haus mit einem Freund teilten. Wir führten dort sechs Monate lang ein glückliches Leben, dann brauchte die Vermieterin unsere Zimmer, und so mussten wir wieder umziehen.

Harry verließ Hawaii, um in Österreich ein neues Leben zu beginnen, und daher zogen Serena und ich in seine Wohnung, eine wunderschöne Eigentumswohnung am Golfplatz von Wailea, die er mit Mirra Rose geteilt hatte. Er hatte das Landhaus kurze Zeit nach uns verlassen, da die Miete erhöht worden war und Mirra ein Zimmer frei hatte und einen Mitbewohner suchte. Dies war wieder einmal ein göttliches Timing. Mirra öffnete ihre Wohnung und ihr Herz und bat uns herein, es fühlte sich wunderbar an, und alles war in göttlicher Ordnung. Wir verbrachten sogar Harrys letzte zehn Tage gemeinsam und erlebten eine schöne Zeit miteinander, bevor er wegging. Wir alle liebten das Zusammenleben, hatten eine Menge Spaß und halfen uns gegenseitig. Unglücklicherweise war dies nur von kurzer Dauer, da wir Maui verlassen mussten, um uns nach England zu begeben und ein Studentenvisum für Serena zu beantragen, die im Herbst wieder zurückkommen und mit dem Studium beginnen wollte. Gegen Ende Mai 2003 verließ ich Maui schließlich als Einwohnerin.

Ich war ausgesprochen traurig, doch ich wusste, dass dies der nächste Schritt war. Mutter Maui war mir in einer Meditation erschienen und hatte mir gesagt, dass ich ein Küken in ihrem Nest war und dass es nun an der Zeit für mich sei, wegzufliegen. Und wenn ich das nicht tun würde, würde sie mich aus dem Nest stoßen! Sie sagte mir, dass es für mich an der Zeit sei, meine Geschenke und alles, was ich auf diesem Weg der Selbsterkenntnis gelernt hatte, mit der Welt zu teilen.

Wir kamen in England an und wurden von meiner Schwester begrüßt, bei der wir die ersten paar Tage verbrachten. Es war für uns alle eine wunderbare Zusammenkunft, da wir uns seit Jahren nicht mehr gesehen hatten. Wir begaben uns dann zum Haus meiner Eltern in Cornwall, das seit dieser Zeit mein Hauptwohnsitz ist. Wir verbrachten drei glückliche Monate mit meiner Familie, fanden wieder eine Beziehung zueinander und genossen es, in deren Gesellschaft zu sein. Wir erhielten an der amerikanischen Botschaft in London ein Studentenvisum für Serena, und sie kehrte Mitte August nach Maui zurück, um mit dem Studium zu beginnen.

Ich war wieder einmal extrem traurig und einsam, denn mein Baby hatte mich verlassen, und es wurde so schnell erwachsen! Ich begann, mich wieder als Opfer meiner Situation zu fühlen, als mir der geliebte Christus zu Hilfe kam und ein ernstes Wörtchen zu mir sprach! Er fragte mich, was ich in meinem Leben erreichen wollte. Wohin ich gehen und was ich tun wollte. Er sagte, dass es an mir liege, zu entscheiden, was ich mit meinem Leben anfangen wollte. Ich sollte meine Ziele und Visionen aufschreiben und damit beginnen, sie zu manifestieren, anstatt mich elend zu fühlen und Mitleid mit mir zu haben. Dieses innerliche Gespräch, das ich auch schriftlich festgehalten habe, half mir enorm. Es gab mir wieder einmal zu verstehen, dass ich die Verantwortung für mein Leben übernehmen musste und dass es an mir lag, was ich daraus machen wollte, und dass dafür nur ich selbst verantwortlich bin!

Ich schrieb meine Ziele auf, hörte auf, mich als Opfer zu fühlen, und plötzlich tat sich alles auf. Veranstalter aus Europa kontaktierten mich und luden mich ein, nach Deutschland, Österreich und Frankreich zu kommen. Damit überwand ich meine Traurigkeit darüber, Serena verloren zu haben, weil ich mit der Vorbereitung der Seminare beschäftigt war, und dies war ein großer Segen. Ich war von August bis November drei Monate lang in Europa unterwegs, veranstaltete Seminare zum Thema Loslassen von alten Mustern und Gelübden und BioGenesis und führte private Sitzungen durch. Das Seminar an diesem Wochenende trägt den Titel „Der Weg nach Vorne", und es geht darum, unsere Herzen zu öffnen, und alle alten Muster loszulassen, mehr Liebe aufnehmen zu können, die Verantwortung für unser Leben zu übernehmen und zu entscheiden, was wir erreichen möchten, und dabei unsere Macht wieder anzunehmen. Es geht tatsächlich um den Prozess, den ich vor kurzem durchgemacht habe: Das Universum versetzt mich in einen Lernprozess, und dann werde ich hinausgesandt, um anderen das beizubringen, was ich gerade gelernt habe, und das funktioniert wunderbar!

Während ich im Jänner 2004 dieses Kapitel korrigiere, muss ich über die Lektion lachen, die ich soeben durchgemacht habe. Ich habe im Sommer 2003 viele Monate dafür verwendet, in Workshops und Sitzungen alte Gelübde von mir selbst und anderen aufzulösen. Ich schätze, ich musste erfahren, wie mächtig die Worte sind, die wir aussprechen und schreiben, und das auch anderen beibringen. Sie sagen, dass man anderen das beibringt, was man selbst am dringendsten lernen muss, und das stimmte mit Sicherheit! Was ich erkannte, war, dass ich die Gelübde, die ich auf Maui an Gott abgelegt hatte, noch nicht aufgelöst hatte und dass ich mich an die Arbeit machen und sie auflösen musste. Ich hatte solche Angst davor, einen Fehler zu begehen und Gott zu enttäuschen. Ich wollte auf jeden Fall weiterhin dienen, so gut ich es konnte, und wollte keinen Rückzieher von meiner Verpflichtung gegenüber Gott machen und mich auch nicht von meiner Beziehung zu Gott distanzieren.

Trotz meiner Angst hatte ich das Gefühl, dass es das Richtige war. Am nächsten Tag, während einem BioGenesis-Seminar, das ich abhielt, löste ich die Gelübde mit Hilfe von Gundi auf, und es war ein wunderbares Gefühl, sie aufzulösen! Ich forderte meine Macht zurück und hatte eine riesige Lektion gemeistert. Ich war so damit beschäftigt, anderen beim Auflösen der alten Gelübde zu helfen, dass ich dabei meine eigenen Gelübde ganz vergessen hatte. Die große Lektion lautete: Verschenke

Deine Macht nicht mehr an jedermann! Gott befindet sich nicht außerhalb von uns selbst, sondern in jedem von uns. Gott ist im Leben in allem gegenwärtig. Diese allwissende Weisheit und Liebe, die wir Gott nennen, ist in jeder Zelle unseres Körpers, in allem, was existiert, gegenwärtig. Alles, was wir zu tun haben, besteht darin, in jeder Minute jedes Tages von dieser mächtigen ICH-BIN-Gegenwart im Inneren geführt zu werden.

Wir legen auch viele unbewusste Gelübde in unserem täglichen Leben ab und erkennen nicht, wie mächtig diese sind. Um frei zu werden, ist es erforderlich, auch diese Versprechungen aufzugeben. Im Laufe der Zeit werden wir weiser und verstehen sämtliche Lernerfahrungen, die wir durchgemacht haben. Wir sind hier, um zu lernen, und das tun wir auch mit Sicherheit auf die eine oder andere Weise. Das Universum ist vollkommen organisiert. Alles, was wir lernen müssen, kommt immer wieder zurück, bis wir die Lektion schließlich begreifen! Dann können wir wahrlich dankbar sein für alles, was in unserem Leben geschehen ist und uns der Meisterschaft einen Schritt näher gebracht hat.

Die wichtigsten Gelübde sind:

a) Armutsgelübde und Gelübde,
   die das Materielle ablehnen (Wurzelchakra)

b) Keuschheitsgelübde und Gelübde sexueller Abstinenz (Sakralchakra)

c) Gelübde der Selbstaufopferung und Selbstverleugnung (Solarplexus)

d) Zölibat und Gelübde des Getrenntseins (Herzchakra)

e) Schweigegelübde und Gelübde der vorsätzlichen Verleugnung (Kehlkopfchakra)

f) Gelübde des Leidens und der Vergeltung (Chakra des dritten Auges)

g) Gelübde des Gehorsams und der Demut (Kronenchakra)

Falls Sie Ihrem Gefühl nach Gelübde aus einem vergangenen oder gegenwärtigen Leben haben, können Sie diese mit einigen einfachen Schritten auflösen. Gelübde werden von einem Leben ins nächste übertragen, sofern sie nicht bewusst auf diese Weise aufgelöst werden. Als ich mit dieser Arbeit begann, konnte jeweils nur ein Gelübde auf einmal aufgelöst werden. Jetzt habe ich festgestellt, dass es in all meinen Sitzungen gestattet ist, sämtliche Gelübde auf einmal aufzulösen. Versuchen Sie es selbst, und Sie werden wissen, was für Sie richtig ist. Es ist wichtig, das Muster, das durch dieses Gelübde verursacht wurde, zu erkennen und es bewusst loszulassen.

1. Reinigen Sie sich vor und nach diesem Prozess in der Dusche oder in einem Vollbad.

2. Trinken Sie vorher und nachher jede Menge Wasser.

3. Legen Sie sich hin und machen Sie es sich bequem.

4. Verbinden Sie sich mit Ihrem höheren Selbst, der Gottesgegenwart in Ihrem Herzen.

5. Bitten Sie die Meister und Engel, Sie bei diesem Loslösungsprozess zu unterstützen.

6. Bitten Sie darum, dass Ihnen die Gelübde gezeigt werden, die Sie auflösen sollen.

7. Wenn Ihnen klar ist, welche Gelübde Sie auflösen sollen, bitten Sie darum, dass Ihnen gezeigt werden möge, was Sie daraus gelernt haben. Wie Sie diese Gelübde am Leben erhalten und ihnen gedient haben. Bedanken Sie sich bei den Gelübden für alles, was Sie gelernt haben, und bereiten Sie sich darauf vor, sie loszulassen.

8. Umgeben Sie Ihren gesamten Körper oder das entsprechende Chakra mit einer riesigen golde-

nen, heilenden Lichtkugel und wiederholen Sie die folgenden Sätze laut und aus tiefstem Herzen.

9. In der Vergangenheit habe ich ein Gelübde der/des .... abgelegt. Ich habe aus diesem Gelübde viel gelernt. (Sprechen Sie nun laut aus, was Sie gelernt haben.) In der Gegenwart und für die Zukunft erkenne ich allerdings, dass mir dieses alte Gelübde der/des .... nicht mehr länger dienlich ist. Ich lasse dieses alte Gelübde aus meinem Energiefeld, meinem Körper und meinem Bewusstsein, auf allen Ebenen und Dimensionen, los. Und damit auch sämtliche Beschränkungen, die dadurch in meinem Leben verursacht wurden. Ich gehe nun ein neues Versprechen ein (Armut wird durch Fülle ersetzt, Keuschheit durch Schöpfung, Selbstverleugnung durch Eigenliebe, Trennung durch Einheit, Stille durch Ausdruck, Leiden durch freudvolles Leben und Gehorsam durch Vertrauen) und integriere es in mein Wesen. Ich bitte meine Geistführer, die neuen Energien dieses Versprechens nun in mein Leben einzubringen. Ich nehme das neu Erlernte und die wundersamen Veränderungen, die dieses neue Versprechen mit sich bringen wird, an. So sei es, so ist es.

10. Wenn Sie damit fertig sind, beseitigen Sie die alte Energie aus den Zellen Ihres Körpers und führen

Sie diese in die goldene heilende Lichtkugel. Rufen Sie die mächtige violette Flamme an, um in Ihren vier niederen Körpern sowie rund um diese herum zu brennen, Aufzeichnungen und Erinnerungen, Ursache und Wirkung dieses alten Gelübdes zu reinigen und zu säubern. Bitten Sie dann die Engel, Ihren gesamten Körper mit einem laserartigen Lichtstrahl zu reinigen, und gehen Sie sicher, dass die ganze alte Energie verschwunden ist. Dann übergeben Sie die goldene heilende Kugel an den universellen Lebensstrom und lassen Sie alles los!

Der Großteil unserer alten Muster ist in gewisser Weise mit den Gelübden verbunden, die wir in der Vergangenheit abgelegt haben, und daher besteht das einzige, was Sie zu tun haben, darin, Ihr Leben zu betrachten. Wenn Sie sich die Muster und Glaubenssätze, die Sie haben, ansehen, werden Sie bald wissen, welche Gelübde Sie aufzulösen haben.

Das Universum hat mir ein Ticket mit Freimeilen für Maui geschenkt, und dafür bin ich wirklich dankbar und überglücklich! Ich werde also am 20. Februar 2004 zurückkehren, um die Mädchen, meine Freunde und Mutter Maui zu besuchen. Ich freue mich auch schon darauf, wieder bei meinen Kindern sein zu können, denn ich vermisse sie. In dieser Zeit werde ich für eine Reisegruppe aus Europa gemeinsam mit Mirra Rose eine magische Reisetour veranstalten und an den heiligen Orten Seminare abhalten. Ich habe die Absicht, jedes Jahr eine Gruppe nach Maui zu begleiten und die Schätze der Insel mit ihnen zu teilen. Es ist stets eine lebensverändernde Erfahrung für jeden, die er nie mehr vergessen wird.

Ich habe während meiner Reisen eine Menge gelernt. Da ich keinen festen Aufenthaltsort habe, ist dieses Leben ein wenig anders als das, welches ich einst gewohnt war. Ich habe festgestellt, dass ich überall glücklich sein kann, und mein wirkliches Zuhause befindet sich in meinem Herzen. Die Zeit, in der ich zuhause bei meinen Eltern lebte, war sehr kostbar, da ich auch Zeit mit meiner Mutter verbringen konnte, die nicht mehr so beweglich ist und die ich in den letzten dreißig Jahren nicht sehr oft gesehen hatte. Alles ist in göttlicher Ordnung. Ich freue mich auf jeden Tag und frage mich, was das Universum für mich bereithalten wird. Ich empfinde in meinem Herzen einen tiefen Frieden und Glückseligkeit, obwohl ich in meinem Leben außer einigen Kleidungsstücken, Schmuck, einem Laptop und einem Telefon nichts Materielles besitze. Die Lebensfreude ist in meinem Herzen, und ich nehme diese Freude mit, wohin auch immer ich gehe. Ich arbeite noch daran, die tiefe Traurigkeit in meinem Herzen zu heilen, die mich überkommt, wenn ich meine geliebte Heimat Maui verlassen muss, doch ich weiß, dass auch dies irgendwann geheilt sein wird, denn je mehr ich mein Herz öffne, desto mehr werde ich von innen heraus geheilt!

Dies war eine kurze Beschreibung meines Lebens mit all seinen Höhen und Tiefen der vergangenen Jahre. Ich hoffe, dass dies einigen von Ihnen in Zeiten von Problemen und Verzweiflung helfen wird, zu verstehen, dass der Prozess, den Sie durchmachen, wahrhaftig göttlicher Art ist und dass Sie einfach nur alles, was in Ihrem Leben passiert, akzeptieren und annehmen sollen, anstatt es zu bekämpfen. Wenn Sie die Umstände akzeptieren und sie dem höheren Selbst übergeben, wird sich der göttliche Plan entfalten. Das Leben ist mit Sicherheit eine Aufgabe, die sich im Inneren abspielt, und der Weg ist das Ziel!

Kümmern Sie sich gut um sich selbst, und lassen Sie sich von der Liebe in Ihrem Herzen führen. Leben Sie jeden Augenblick im Glück, und machen Sie sich keine Sorgen um die Zukunft.

Gott segne Sie alle!

Nachwort

Achtet auf Eure Gedanken, verurteilt Euch selbst oder andere nicht. Beobachtet die Gedanken, liebt sie und vergebt ihnen und sendet sie hinaus.

Ihr seid getarnte Meister – liebt diese Tarnung, und Ihr werdet Eure Meisterschaft entdecken. Niemand ist unfähig, diese Wahrheit zu erkennen, es ist nur so, dass Ihr diese Fähigkeit manchmal vergessen habt!

Euer Prozess ist vollkommen, selbst wenn Ihr diese Vollkommenheit nicht ausdrücken könnt. Ihr solltet dies vom Standpunkt Eures höheren Selbst aus verstehen. Durch das Spiel an sich wird der Sieg eingebracht und die Freude gefunden.

Ihr werdet Fehler begehen, doch Ihr seid Meister und Ihr werdet einen Weg finden. Dabei solltet Ihr Eure eigenen Fehler mit derselben Vergebung beobachten, die auch ein Kind von seinen Eltern erhält. Bringt Euch selbst dieselbe Liebe entgegen.

Wenn Ihr Eure Fehler, die Ganzheit Eures Seins, totale Vergebung und das Loslassen sämtlicher alter Muster annehmt, wird Vollkommenheit erlangt.

Arbeitet daran, Euren Glauben und Sonnenschein in Eurem Herzen zu bewahren, und strahlt dieses Licht der Wahrheit aus, das nicht verleugnet werden kann. Die Meisterschaft war den langen und dunklen Tunnel der Verzweiflung wert.

In der vollkommenen Verwirklichung dieser Schlüssel liegt eine Freiheit, eine Freude und eine Leichtigkeit. Die Leichtigkeit eines Kindes, die erst dann wirklich erkannt werden kann, wenn zu allen Zeiten, in jedem Augenblick in der Vergangenheit, Gegenwart und Zukunft, eine Verpflichtung und eine vollkommene Vergebung präsent sind. Mit dieser Verpflichtung werdet Ihr keinen Schaden zu sehen bekommen und auch niemandem Schaden zufügen. Die Wahrheit wird offenbart, denn Eure Worte können nur die Wahrheit aussprechen, Eure Handlungen können nur Liebe geben, und diese Verpflichtung setzt die volle Macht Eurer ICH-BIN-GEGENWART frei.

Gebet für die Vollkommenheit

Das eine Wesen ist ganz und vollkommen.

Daher bin ich ganz und vollkommen.

Und alles ist ein Teil von mir

und Ich bin ein Teil von allem.

Es kann keine Fehler geben,

und auch nichts zu vergeben, wenn alles eins ist.

Ich bin eins mit diesem Einen WESEN,

und indem ich alles annehme,

rufe ich die Ganzheit der Vollkommenheit,

das Wissen und die reine Wahrheit an.

Bei diesem Gebet geht es darum, um die Ganzheit der Vollkommenheit und um die Vollkommenheit der Ganzheit zu bitten.